Simple Secrets to Easy Weight Loss

The diet free and pain free
Weight Management System
designed for your lifestyle of today.

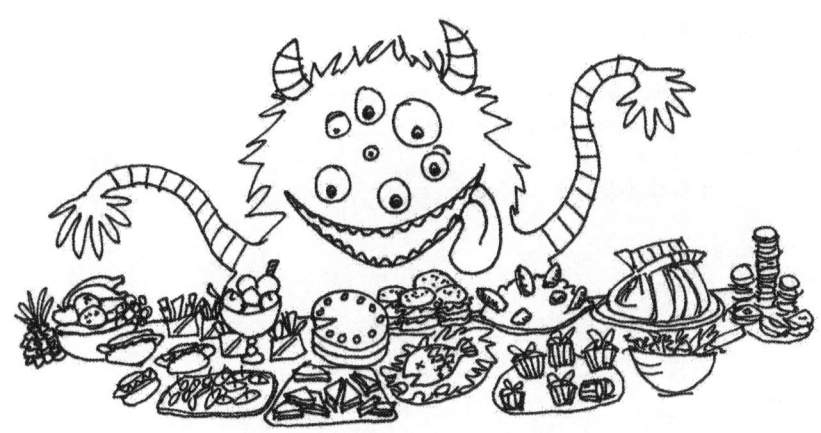

Steve McNulty

With an exciting and valuable introduction to
Thought Field Therapy®
by the creator of TFT, Dr Roger Callahan

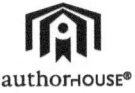

authorHOUSE®

AuthorHouse™ UK Ltd.
500 Avebury Boulevard
Central Milton Keynes, MK9 2BE
www.authorhouse.co.uk
Phone: 08001974150

First published by AuthorHouse   9/12/2007

ISBN: 978-1-4343-3066-6 (sc)

Printed in the United States of America
Bloomington, Indiana

This book is printed on acid-free paper.

Welcome

Eating is one of life's great pleasures and I want you to enjoy eating every time you eat. Hunger is the body's way of telling us we need food and this is a critical protection function of our natural system. Therefore, you will never go hungry using my specially designed and developed Oh-Crikey techniques.

My weight management technique uses every thing and every technique I have found to work and uses none of the fads or deprivation diets we all know do not really work. I will teach you a pain free, craving free, deprivation free, hunger free, surgery free, drug free, supplement free, anxiety free, easy to understand and easy to follow set of guidelines that, if followed reasonably closely (yes, you are allowed to lapse occasionally), will help you manage your weight successfully.

More importantly, it will help you manage your weight at the level you decide is right for you and will help you feel good about yourself, improve your confidence and put more control back in your life. It is important to state right at the start that this is not a diet, diets do not work. This is also not strict or demanding and doesn't require lots of willpower or memory.

My weight management system is based on the causes and reasons why we eat when we are not hungry and shows you easy ways to eliminate the anxiety and associated cravings. It allows you to set the pace, set the levels and set the results.

It is the only system I know of that puts you in total control of your weight. Why is it revolutionary? Because it takes all the things we have known for centuries e.g. eat when you are hungry, chew your food well, stop when you are full etc and then adds the easy to use and powerful 21st Century therapy for addictions and cravings (Thought Field Therapy), created and developed by Dr Roger Callahan.

This includes an understanding of Individual Energy Toxins and which makes a significant difference to helping you achieve success.

I developed this system while I was losing weight and I wanted to ensure that I did it consistently and that it was permanent. I love my food and enjoy eating, so it had to fit in with that. I lost 42 pounds in 18 months whilst eating as much as I wanted, when I wanted it. I believe fully that it will work for you in the manner you decide fits you best.

Steve McNulty

Acknowledgements

I would like to thank Dr Roger Callahan the creator of Callahan Techniques® Thought Field Therapy® (TFT). Without his life-long perseverance in trying to continually find new and better ways to help people eliminate suffering, we would not have TFT.

Without TFT, many people around the world would be suffering unnecessarily, there would be a lot more pain in the world and I would not be managing my weight successfully. The techniques used in 'The Secret to Easy Weight Loss' incorporate many of Dr Callahan's very successful processes and treatments. He has very kindly written the Foreword to this book and also a great introduction to TFT and this can be found in Appendix 1.

My thanks go to Paul McKenna for helping me start my quest to lose weight when he trained me in Neuro Linguistic Programming (NLP).

All my family and colleagues deserve my thanks for supporting and encouraging me throughout the complete process.

Thanks go to Jack Vincent, Sandra Wilson, Jackie Gibbins, Joanne Callahan, Colin Davies, my wife and Chief Editor Elaine, my sister Geraldine, my brother Martin and all my friends for encouraging and assisting me. Your help was invaluable.

Foreword

In 2005, Steve, at 54 years old, decided that if he didn't start to control his weight he would face significant health issues in later life. He had previously tried all varieties of system but none would fit into how he wanted to live his life. He made a commitment to develop a system that would suit him and many millions of people like him.

During Steve's quest for the 'holy grail' of weight management systems, he searched for techniques and methods that would provide all the positive elements that he wanted for himself such as losing weight, getting fitter, feeling better and looking better. He wanted these benefits without the normally associated negative consequences such as deprivation, supplements, diets, excessive exercise, rigid regimes, drugs, surgery, fads, etc. In fact, he wanted everything without having to pay for it. He wanted to be able to control his weight while living and thoroughly enjoying the modern lifestyle of a successful businessman.

The system in this book is the fruition of Steve's work. He is proof of its ability to make a significant difference. Steve is now 42 pounds lighter than he was 18 months ago and he is fitter, healthier and happier than he was in his thirties. His students are now reaping the benefit of this system.

He started off with everything his Mother and other adults told him when he was a child. Things like don't go hungry – if you are hungry eat something; chew your food properly; eat slowly – it's not a race; don't eat between meals – have a drink of water etc. He then added elements of exercise management (without the effort) he had learned from years as a sportsman. Adding to this mind management techniques he learned from training in NLP and Hypnotherapy and finally a good sprinkling of common sense.

This system worked but it was missing something that would make it really special and I am proud to say that Steve found it the therapy I created, Thought Field Therapy®.

Steve was and still is a student of mine. He wanted to investigate all the reasons why we eat when we are not hungry; what are the causes and effects; is there a basic reason behind all overeating; what we can do to stop doing this; how we can stop food addiction cravings without pain and similar questions. Steve found the answers to all these questions and more in his study of TFT.

By adding TFT as the major critical success factor to his Weight Management System, Steve has created a system that is truly for the 21st Century lifestyle.

I have enjoyed advising Steve in the production of this book and the associated course.

If you follow his guidelines you have every chance to live your life to the full and still control your weight effectively.

Dr Roger Callahan
Creator of Thought Field Therapy®

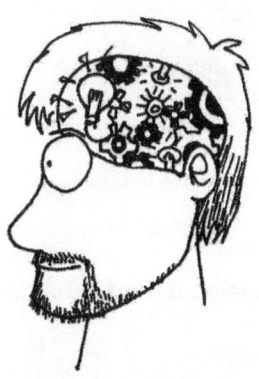

Chapters

Preface

My aim in writing this book is to set you free. To give you the freedom to do what **you** want to do. To give you the techniques that will help you manage or be free of external controlling influences. This applies not only to weight issues but also to other areas of your life.

When we are unable to stop eating, even when we are not hungry, it means we are addicted to food. All addictions, great and small, I believe are caused by anxiety, and all addictive substances, including food, are tranquilisers that serve to mask our anxiety.

The reasons that diets, fasting, deprivation and surgery etc don't work is because they treat the symptom rather than the cause. Most, if not all, weight issues are a result of anxiety of one form or another. This anxiety is displayed in a number of ways including boredom, stress, worry, distraction, comfort and so on.

My aim is to give you control over your anxiety, so that you can choose what you want to eat and when you want to eat it. I will also show you how to feel good for absolutely no reason whatsoever without having to eat.

To achieve this there are some basics that you need to work on. They are 1) you really do need to know what you want for the future and 2) you also really do need to know where you are now.

So there are some elements of this book that explore your future hopes and aspirations, and tests your knowledge of where you are currently. All this information is maintained privately to you and your answers and future objectives are known only to you. So if you lie to yourself, the only person you are kidding and hurting is you.

Based on the knowledge you will gain from the early chapters you can decide how free you wish to be and how much control you want to have over your own destiny.

I use a number of techniques in the book to help you. The main and most powerful technique I use by far is Thought Field Therapy® (TFT) created and developed by Dr Roger Callahan. Roger created this amazing therapy 25 years ago and has been developing it ever since. TFT is an accepted complementary therapy to which medical doctors may refer their patients. TFT is accredited by the National Health Service Trust Association (NHS TA).

This TFT process is vitally important in managing your weight and can be achieved by everyone from every walk of life with a little application and a desire to increase their happiness. Relax and enjoy the journey.

Steve McNulty

Chapter 1
Introduction

Congratulations, you have made a great decision to read this book. These guidelines will help you manage your weight at the level you are comfortable with and, more importantly I think, help you to feel good about yourself. I know that you will, quite rightly, take the bits you like and use them and leave anything that doesn't feel quite right to one side. All I ask is that you do everything I ask of you for the first 12 days.

Once you have completed successfully the first 12 days, treat the techniques in here as your own personal strategy. Think of it that way and develop a strategy that works for you but that takes in at least half to three-quarters of my guidelines.

If you do this, I believe that you will be able to manage your weight properly, consistently, easily and at a level that you are happy with.

Remember that, at all times, you can use the techniques you learn here for every area of your life and not just weight issues. You never have to suffer needlessly again.

Learn at your own pace, in your own time and ensure you understand each area before moving on.

It is really important to me that you succeed. You have bought this book because you want to succeed. Therefore, it is safe to say that we both want you to succeed.

Your success is NOT dependent on following religiously everything I say for ever and a day! You are allowed to make mistakes, you are allowed to lapse occasionally.

However, these mistakes or lapses must always have less effect than the effect of doing the right thing. The result will be a slower movement towards controlling your weight.

With the TFT processes will cover, you do not have to believe in the process for it to work. It just does.

If you do what I ask of you in this book, you will have every chance to succeed.

There is a Success Booklet that accompanies this book. For your copy register with us at www.oh-crikey.com and you will be able to download your personal copy. Once you have read the programme, review it and write all your plans and objectives in your success booklet. Use the booklet daily for encouragement and as a guide to your progress.

Chapter 2
The Principles of Weight Management

Overweight or underweight – according to whom

Have you ever seen catwalk models, film stars, pop stars etc in real life? Have you ever been amazed at how different they look in real life, without the 'airbrushing', photographic effects or make up?

The alterations made to photographs before publication compromise reality in order to fit the media's view of what is the perfect shape/ weight/hair cut/ shoe shape/etc. The images are not real but many people aspire to be as unreal and they can never achieve it. That is, unless they have access to the entire make up artists and photographers assistants that are available to the media. So let's stop trying to be someone else and let's start being ourselves.

Who decides whether you are overweight or underweight? There should be only two arbiters of this. The first is YOU and the second is your doctor. If your doctor says your weight is affecting your health, you should listen and do something about it.

Otherwise, it is up to you where you feel most comfortable in terms of your weight. I have large and small friends who would not be the people they are if their weight changed dramatically. They are comfortable with themselves and their weight and they are happy.

My techniques will put you in control of your weight and bring contentment and happiness. Remember – **you** decide everything for you.

You are not broken, you don't need to be fixed – all you need are some selected techniques to put you back in control.

Weight Loss v Weight Management

I don't want you to lose weight for the sake of losing weight. I want you to be able to control your weight at the level that makes you feel the best about every bit of you.

Therefore, I prefer to talk about and teach techniques for weight management.

Weight management is all about deciding what weight level suits you. It also helps decide on weight issues as we grow older and less active.

Weight and weight management are not cast in stone. The criteria changes whenever you feel it is appropriate that they change.

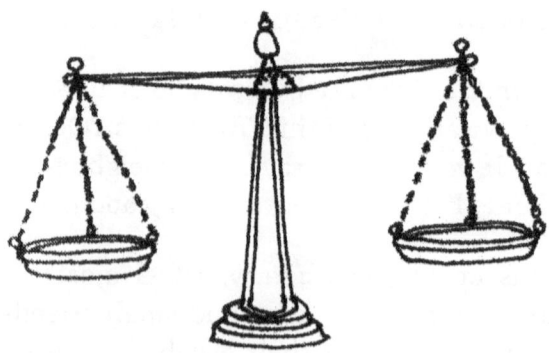

Eating v Exercise – the balance

We are always told that the simplest way to lose weight is eat less and exercise more. Alternatively, to put weight on you should exercise less and eat more.

However, the more sportspeople exercise, the heavier they get. Why? Muscle is heavier than fat. So do we want to lose weight or lose fat? Do we want to be thin or muscular? Do we want to be athletes or just basically fit? We want what we want and not what someone else thinks we should have – right?

Well, let's be reasonable about this. We want to control our weight and our looks so that we have the right balance of healthy and pleasurable eating with a level of exercise that keeps us fit. We want to look how we want to look and how we feel comfortable with ourselves, but at the same time that doesn't require us to maintain muscle levels or unpleasant exercise regimes.

I will work with you to provide you with the techniques to produce what you want and not what someone else perceives as correct. Remember, the airbrushed models are not real.

Why we eat

There are many reasons why we eat when we do and why we eat what we eat. Some of the more common ones are covered below

Hunger

We start at the obvious reason – hunger. We must eat in order to live. Hunger is our body's sign to tell us that we need energy. Energy is taken in the form of food.

However, many of us mistake thirst for hunger. Our lifestyles and environment mean that we lose fluid quicker now than at any time in the past. The pangs of dehydration are similar to hunger and cause the same reaction. However, we tend to go straight to food as the solution. We can and will learn how to use liquid, and especially water, as a 'snack' to help us fight off the 'phantom' hunger pangs.

Try a glass of water, cup of tea or coffee when you think you are hungry and see if the hunger feelings go away. If they don't – then you need to eat. If they do, then you don't need to eat.

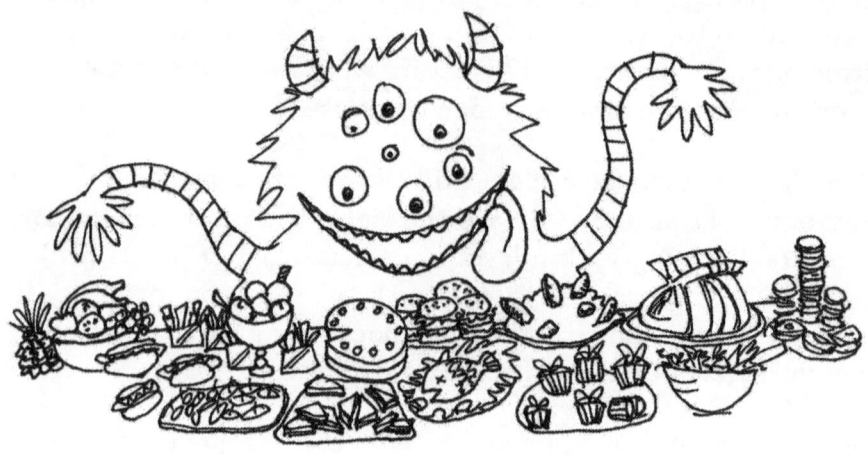

Enjoyment

There no doubt that eating can be one of the great enjoyments in life. It is certainly one of my great pastimes. My friends cannot believe how I can 'Eat for England' and still manage my weight effectively.

An earthy bouillabaisse, the perfect sausage and mash, paella, Quattro formaggio pizza, penne arrabiata, mom's meat loaf, apple and blueberry pie, a full English breakfast, a short stack of pancakes with maple syrup and many more are all great to taste and enjoy.

Wherever you are in the world, whatever your favourite food, why should you have to go without? Why should you deprive yourself? You need not. Yes – you can eat your favourite food – even chocolate.

I want you to enjoy fully everything you eat. No exceptions at all. No reason to put junk in your mouth. Everything we eat, we eat because we really enjoy it.

Emotion

The way we feel plays a very big part in why and how we eat. Below are some of the common emotional eating triggers:

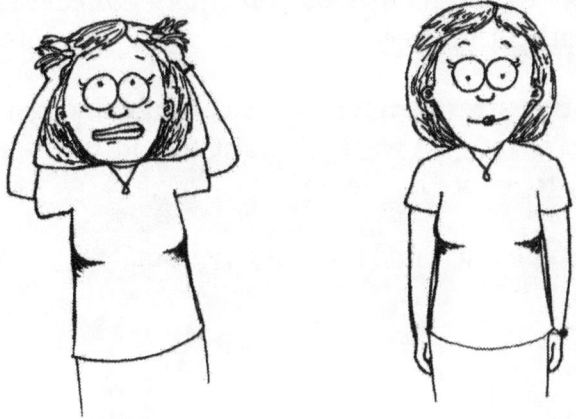

Stress

There are only four ways to reduce stress. One, take away the reason to be stressed. Two, take medication to make you forget about the stress. Three, distract yourself with something else, and four, choose not to be stressed.

Reaching for your de-stressing food and, in fact any food, does help you reduce your stress but only because it distracts you from the stressful issue. In fact, it masks the stress based anxiety.

It changes the way you feel, but only temporarily. We can do this much more easily and quickly and with no harmful effects.

When you eat to mask the anxiety symptoms of stress, the food itself will help increase your heart rate and blood pressure. So food in its own right can increase the stress on your body's systems but it can also distract you from a stressful situation.

Reaching for food in a stressful situation quickly becomes a habit. So we have the double issue of habit and distraction adding to our loss of control. You then become addicted to the food and this just adds to the issue.

I will show you how to use options three and four above, without forming negative habits or food addictions, to reduce stress and, therefore, without the need to reach for the food comforter.

It is proven that stress can lead to weight gain amongst other non-healthy side effects. So we don't want to add to the problem by eating to try to reduce it – do we?

We will treat the cause and not the symptom.

Boredom

If you decide to chill out and do nothing for 30 minutes, close your eyes and rest – are you bored? Of course not. If you have 30 minutes on your hands with nothing to do – are you bored? Probably. What's the difference? The difference is the anxiety you feel because you should be doing something and you are not. So we try to change the way we feel and we reach for food.

Reaching for food because we are bored is, again, a distraction.

When we are really interested in something and concentrating on it to the exclusion of everything else, we often forget to eat and even forget to drink? How often do you deliberately stop to eat when you are really busy and really engrossed in something?

I will show you how to use our techniques, without forming negative habits, to reduce boredom and, therefore, the need to reach for the food comforter.

Let's treat the cause and not the symptom.

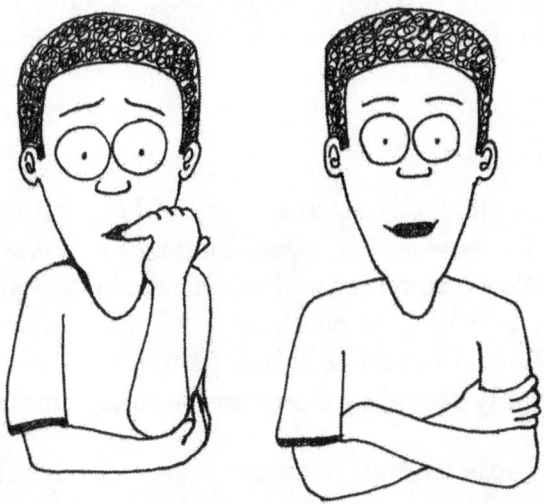

Anxiety

Anxiety is a type of fear that is pervasive, unfocused and extremely unpleasant. Anxiety is the partner of stress. The need to mask the feelings of anxiety is, I believe, the cause of addiction. In other words, no anxiety no addiction.

Some anxiety is good and forms part of our protection systems. Also sports people tell us that they need an amount of anxiety in order to perform at their peak. They call it 'The Edge' or 'The Zone'. However, most sportsmen would rate this as a low level of anxiety that carries no harmful stress with it.

Anxiety causes our food addiction just as it causes irrational fear in phobics. However, there is one important difference: where a phobic can point to something specific as the source of his or her phobia (e.g. bridges, spiders etc) the food addict is usually not that specific. You may not be even conscious of having anxiety.

I will show you how to use the techniques for anxiety elimination, without forming negative habits, to reduce it and, therefore, the need to reach for the food comforter.

Comfort

We often hear people tell us that eating provides them with comfort feelings. You know what – it does. The process of eating requires the body to release enzymes and chemicals. These can provide us with temporary feelings of pleasure and comfort. But…. yes, what we are doing is masking the feelings of anxiety. We are not treating the cause but only providing a temporary change in feelings.

You can have those feelings without eating! Yes – it's true.

I will show you how.

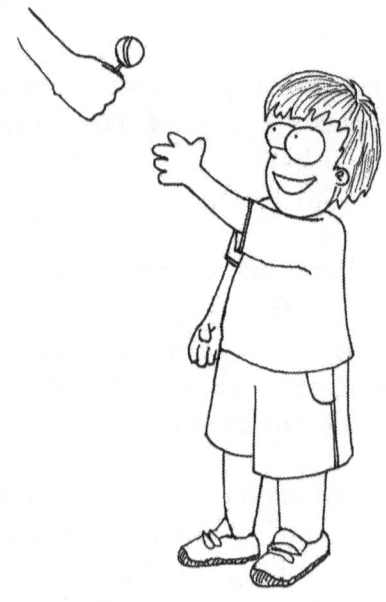

Reward

If you are a good little person I will reward you with a special treat. How often were we told this as a child? How often was this special treat an apple? Or was it more likely to be a chocolate bar?

In later life we then tend to reward ourselves with a treat of high sugar, high salt food.

We need to alter our reward system to something more beneficial. I will show you how.

Substitute

Some people eat more than they need as a substitute habit for something else. For example, people giving up smoking can put on weight due to excessive eating. They blame eating as a substitute for smoking.

I am baffled as to why eating would provide the same effect as smoking for them. Well, it doesn't. After 48 – 72 hours all the nicotine in a smoker's system has disappeared. The only thing left is a habit, or for some the even the worse phenomenon of psychological addiction. The habit and distraction of having a cigarette is replaced with a habit and distraction of eating. Habit, habit, habit. Some people can develop a psychological addiction to certain foods. If this is you, I will show you how to break this.

Now we have two real reasons to eat (hunger and enjoyment) and six other reasons why we eat when we are not hungry. In fact, I would like to add one more social reason and one more psychological reason.

Sociability

When we have guests or we are a guest, invariably there is food available. Even just popping in for a cup of tea or coffee we are served biscuits, cakes, nibbles etc. A great part of social life is eating out either at someone else's house or in a restaurant.

Why should this have to change? It doesn't have to. I want you to enjoy eating. It is one of life's great pleasures.

What I want is for you to choose what you eat, when you eat it and most of all that you enjoy it fully.

You don't have to eat to be sociable, so choose what you want to do and when.

Habit

Understanding how the Mind works is essential in developing great eating and exercise habits. Yes, we want to develop habits because some habits are good for us. Think of some good habits and some bad habits like brushing our teeth or smoking.

The unconscious mind cannot distinguish between good and bad habits because everything our mind does, unconsciously, it does for a good reason. Even with smoking! So for simple habits we just need to remember for a while until it sinks into our unconscious.

If we do something enough times in a short period, the unconscious mind stores it as a habit and we then do not have to think consciously about it. Take driving a car for example. When we first start to drive we have to think about loads of different things in order to control the car. Now we do it without thinking. All habits are the same. For smokers, 20 cigarettes a day for 20 years is over 140,000 cigarettes. Enough times I would say to develop a strong habit.

Ask 1,000 smokers about the experience of smoking their first cigarette and there will be very few who say anything other than it was awful. That is because most people started smoking for one of the following reasons:

- To fit in with their friends
- To look older
- As a rite of passage

These are very valid reasons and your unconscious mind will accept these as good reasons to smoke even if the act of smoking is harming you.

As we get older our reasons for doing things change but unless we tell our unconscious mind that the reasons for the habit are no longer valid it will carry on as if nothing has changed.

Are the above reasons for starting to smoke valid 20 or 30 years on? Probably not. Have smokers told their unconscious mind that it is now not appropriate? Probably not because they fear the consequences (anxiety). The masking of this anxiety creates the addiction.

We develop eating habits and addictions in a similar way and, to break them, we need to understand that there are easier and better ways to achieve the same result without eating.

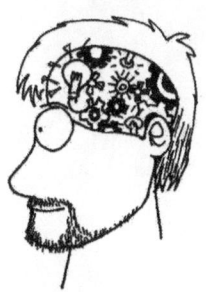

Our unconscious mind is telling us that we need to eat in order to satisfy a requirement set a long time ago. We now need to tell our unconscious mind that the previous good reason for the habit is no longer valid. Once we have done this we can replace the old habit with a new one that is valid for our current needs.

If we are addicted to certain foods we can learn easily how to break this and move forward.

Chapter 3

Why we eat when we are not hungry

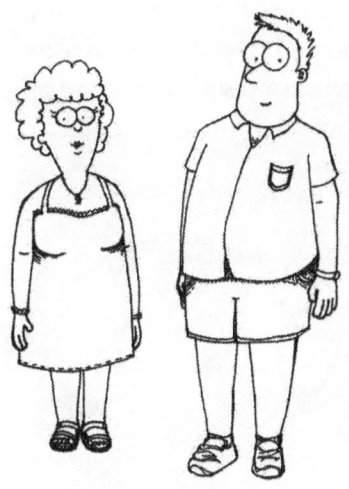

Introduction

So we have a minimum ten reasons to eat. You may be able to add others. Is it no wonder then that we are eating virtually non-stop, with the obvious consequences?

If we could keep hunger as a need to eat, add the enjoyment to it and possibly the social element (once we are control of our weight) we would then have three great reasons to eat.

For the remaining seven unnecessary and unwanted reasons to eat we would need to find other ways to satisfy these emotional requirements the way that eating does. So I am saying that there are seven reasons why we eat when we are not hungry that do not help us in our objectives for weight control. Knowing them means we can control them and eliminate them.

We will do this as we progress through my programme.

First let us examine the reasons and their causes in a bit more depth. The seven unwanted eating processes have been developed over the years by our mind for all the right reasons.

These reasons were formed over the years from childhood and at that time they served a positive purpose. However, they are probably not appropriate now that we are adults. We need to find an adult solution to meeting these needs and develop this into a repeatable habit or process.

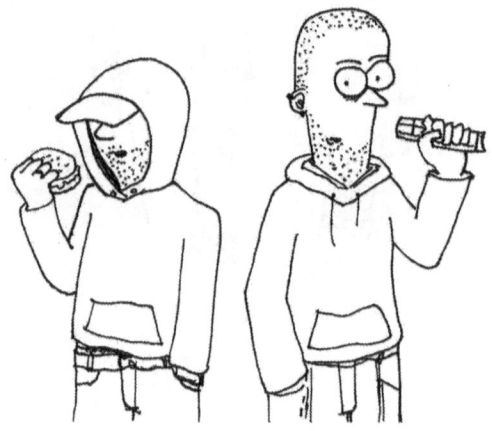

Food addiction

Are you addicted to food? If you do not eat, will you die? Yes, of course. If you do not eat chocolate, will you die? I doubt it very much.

Of course, we need food in order to live. If we were restricted to living on a large farm and all we could find was fruit, vegetables, mushrooms, nuts, river fish and similar items – would we starve?

Of course not! In fact we would have a very healthy eating regime and would have no difficulty in controlling our weight.

Let us say that our favourite food was chocolate. If you had no money would you rob an old lady to get chocolate? If you couldn't get it would you start to have involuntary palpitations and sweating with nausea and withdrawal cramps, just like Heroin? I think not!

We are not addicted to food in a physical reliance way. We are addicted in a psychological way. We can have emotional food reliance. This is a psychological addiction. Psychological addictions have been difficult to shift until now. With the techniques I will show you, you can beat these addictions and replace them with something even better.

Cravings

How often do you say to yourself "I really fancy an apple" or "let's have a salad for tea tonight"? Why don't you do this? Because they don't conjure up feelings you can get from a rapid sugar or salt intake. The so-called healthy options actually provide the level of sugars and salt you need but in a more natural and slower release mode.

Rapid sugar or salt intake can release the chemicals that make you feel great for a short period. So, having felt great for a minute, what do we do? We want to feel good again so we do it again and again and again.

Ready to eat foods are normally high in sugar and fat content and provide a high 'pleasure' effect for the eater.

I will show you how to get over these cravings quickly and easily and without losing any of the benefits.

Habits

Habits are habits. Our unconscious mind does not distinguish between good and bad habits because everything it does, it does for the right reasons. Every habit we have developed over our lifetime started out for the right reasons. This could be to fit in, for protection or to make us feel better.

We explained the smoking habit earlier.

Now, as adults, these reasons may not be appropriate. But have we told our unconscious mind this? Probably not but I will show you how to later on in the programme.

I will show you how, by eliminating your anxiety (known or unknown), you can easily and simply break bad habits and start new good habits.

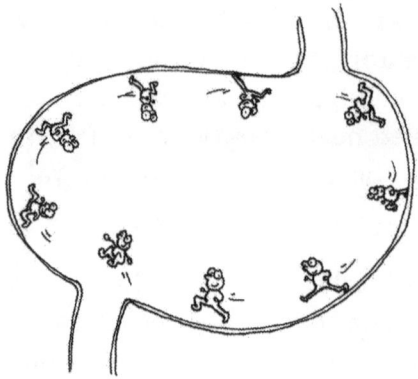

Metabolism

We all have different metabolisms. Your metabolism is the rate that your body burns energy to keep you going. However, our individual metabolism is not static. We can alter it. We can change it permanently.

Some of us are more susceptible to burning off fat due to the nature of our nervous system.

This doesn't mean that we cannot put weight on. The same is due for those of us of a more 'laid back' disposition. This does not mean that we cannot take weight off if we want to.

Chapter 4
Your success contract

We get to the part now that is the start of my simple secrets to easy weight loss. As I said before, some of these have been in existence for centuries and some are revolutionary. The blend of the two produces my system and provides you with the best chance of succeeding in losing weight. But firstly, you must be committed to succeeding.

My commitment to you

I will provide you with everything I know that works for weight management. I will also provide you with techniques that you can take into other areas of your life. I will hold nothing back.

These techniques and methods have worked very well for my students and me, and I am sure that they will work equally well for you.

Once you have read the book and/or taken the course, and I recommend that you do both, I will provide you with an on-line support function and an on-line support group of fellow weight management participants. I will do everything I can to help you succeed in meeting your weight management objectives.

Steve McNulty

Your commitment to yourself

All I ask of you is that you give 100% of your attention, motivation and commitment to achieving your objectives. To do this you will need to follow what I ask exactly for the first 12 days and then you may pick and mix for the remainder in the proportions I advise for the first 12 weeks.

If you do as I ask and you are honest with yourself about it, you will have started towards reaching your objectives after 12 days and will see a significant improvement after 12 weeks.

Are you really ready to manage your weight?

You have heard what I have to say. You know what you want. But.................

Are you really ready to take control of your mind and body and start controlling your weight and feeling better about yourself? Yes?

Great let's go!

What is this weight management technique?

My technique teaches you a pain free, craving free, deprivation free, supplement free, drug free, surgery free, hunger free, easy to understand and easy to follow set of guidelines that, if followed reasonably closely, will help you control your weight.

What does it do for you?

It will give you the opportunity to control your weight at the level that you feel most comfortable with. It will help you feel good about your weight management and help you become happier with your weight.

It does this whilst not stopping you doing anything you really want to stop doing.

You can tie this in with any or all of your future goals and ambitions to help you become the best that you can be.

What you need to do to make it work

Do as I ask for the first 12 days and then at least 50%-75% of what I ask for the remainder of the first 12 weeks. Is that too much to ask for you to get what you want when you want it, every time you want it? No, of course it is not.

There are many good stories of fast weight loss but I want you to lose weight at the rate that suits you. I want you to commit to your personal system that you enjoy using and that will last you a lifetime. I look forward to you being successful.

Chapter 5
Weight management methods and myths

How can we manage our weight?

There are a number of ways we can do this.

It can be slow and painful or long and painful. Which one would you choose? I am joking because it doesn't need to be painful at all. You get to choose the length of time you want to take to achieve your objectives.

Weight management objectives

I consider myself to be part of **your** team. I will be with you and support you every inch of the weigh. Your objectives are my objectives.

You will be doing a bit of writing in this part of the programme and you may be repeating yourself a few times. This is OK so don't worry if you have to repeat yourself – just write down what honestly comes into your mind.

Why do you want to manage your weight?

Write down below why you want to manage your weight. Why **you** really want to. There may be size reasons, health reasons, financial reasons, career reasons, love reasons and others. They are personal to you so be open and honest with yourself.

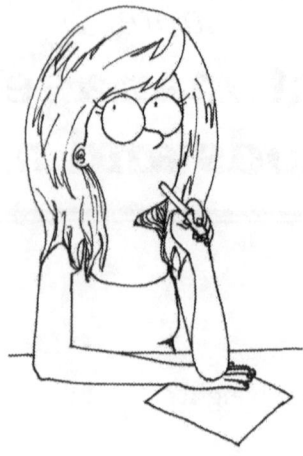

I want to control my weight because:
1
2
3
4
5
6

Write as many as you can. If it is three then stop there. If it is 100 then use a separate piece of paper.

Well done. Look at the reasons. Are they worth achieving?

Three key objectives and 100% commitment

Look at the reasons and make 3 of them key objectives. These should be the ones that will make the biggest improvement to you and your life. These could be things like weigh 12 stone, fit into my old clothes, to walk for 2 miles with my dog, to play with the kids for more than a minute without being out of breath.

I would like you to try to identify one emotional objective e.g. I want to improve my self esteem; one physical objective e.g. I want to be a size 12 and one other which can be another physical or emotional one or another objective e.g. I want to break my reliance on junk food

Write the three key objectives in the left hand column of the table below.

Then in the centre column write down the benefits that achieving it will give to you. For example, if one of the key reasons is to improve your health, then one of the benefits may be to live longer or enjoy holidays more or be able to play with the kids or grandkids properly.

In the right hand column write down how committed you are to achieving this.

Key Objective	Benefits to you	% Commitment

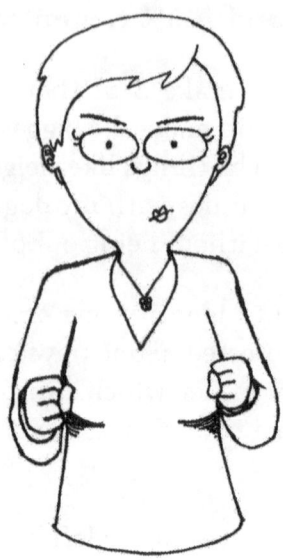

Are you really committed?

Any of the right hand columns above that are not 100% put a line through them and replace them with an objective to which you can commit 100%.

You cannot expect to achieve anything in life unless you are 100% committed.

Don't worry if there is only one objective left. You can achieve this one and then review your overall objectives. If your objective is to reduce your weight to a specific level, let's do that and see what we want to do after we have achieved it.

The objectives above will be turned into specific goals in chapter 6. In chapter 6 we will look at defined and measurable objectives and set reasonable targets so that you can judge your success.

Before I get into specifics let us look at a few of the ideas, methods and myths that are popular components of the weight management arena from time to time.

Methods and Myths

Dieting

Diets do not work. Over 90% of people who diet ultimately fail to lose weight in anything but the short term. Do you really want to lose those pounds only to know that you will put them on again (plus more weight probably) once you stop dieting?

Stop dieting now. Stop using the 'diet' word now. If you are going to be successful following our system, I expressly forbid you to diet in the commonly accepted sense of the word. It doesn't work. It doesn't work. It doesn't work. It doesn't work. Is that enough for you to believe me? 'Diets' do not work with my system.

We have all tried them haven't we? Would you be reading this book if they had worked?

Diets give us all the things we are trying to escape from. They give us hunger, deprivation, anxiety, cravings, pain, upset, fasting, punishment and other negative feelings. Yes, if we are prepared to suffer all the above we may lose weight temporarily but is the short term loss worth the agony of getting there? My system doesn't need pain or agony. You can lose weight permanently with me and have no negative side effects now or in the future.

The aftermath of a failed diet is too horrible to go into here. This cannot happen with my programme because there is no dieting.

So, we don't need diets and we are not allowed to use the word, except in the next two sections.

Temporary dieting

Yo-Yo dieting as it is more commonly known is absolutely no good for you whatsoever. No one has ever succeeded in controlling their weight by binge dieting followed by binge eating.

This is the worst way to try (and fail) to control your weight. It will lead to abject failure and misery. Please don't ever do this.

Permanent dieting

We can think of nothing more soul destroying than being on a permanent diet. These days even Diabetics don't have to be on a restricted diet – just a careful one.

We will not be suggesting that you go on a permanent diet.

Eating less

Eating is a natural and vitally important part of our lives. We have to eat to survive. Hunger is the sign our body gives us so that we know when to eat.

As human beings we are lucky in that we have developed a love for food so that we can enjoy what we eat. Eating can be a great pleasure and we should enjoy it to the full each time we eat.

Now we have two reasons to eat, hunger and enjoyment. These are the two great reasons. I believe that there are no other good reasons to eat, other than sometimes for sociability. All other reasons are a result of negative behaviours, emotions, addictions or habits.

On the scientific side for only a few moments, if you eat less you put less fuel into your body. If you burn up a similar amount of fuel, your body will become weight neutral. If you burn up less than you put in, you will gain weight and if you put in less than you burn up you will lose weight.

Eating less only works to reduce weight if you are burning up more fuel than you are putting in. If you reduce your intake to a level above your burn rate you will still put weight on but only at a slower pace.

We are told about the science of eating less and calorie burning but it doesn't help us with controlling how and why we eat. If we only ate when we were hungry and if we enjoyed fully everything we ate, very few, if any of us would have a weight issue.

Eating less and dieting (sorry to use the word) takes away one of our very important defence systems. It stops us being able to quickly and easily change the way we feel. It stops us getting that temporary respite from the stress of the day.

It stops us being able to mask the feelings of anxiety. So, we don't like it.

We are drawn to masking the feelings of anxiety, even if we don't know we have them.

Also, when you just eat less you will deprive yourself of what you think you need and thereby cause yourself grief. I don't recommend this.

You will eat less with my programme because the reasons for eating when you are not hungry will disappear and you will then eat only because you choose to and when you choose to. You will not realise that you are eating less because you will never be hungry.

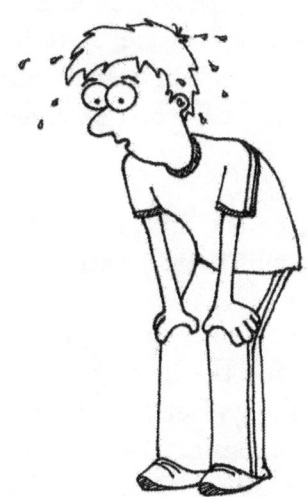

Exercising more

More exercise means burning more calories which means using more fat. It doesn't necessarily mean losing weight.

Exercise can build muscle and muscle is heavier than fat. So excessive exercise can lead to weight gain! Exercise can also tone muscles and provide better body definition.

If our objective is a muscular body with very high definition, then structured and supervised exercise is probably the best way to achieve it. However, I would recommend losing the excess fat first. It is up to you as I want you to manage your weight not necessarily lose weight.

I assume that we all want to reduce our weight, look better and feel better but in a natural way. To achieve this requires us to exercise in a way that is simple, easy and good fun.

You will exercise more with my programme but only in ways that are appropriate to you and at a time of your choosing. This may be an additional short walk a day or a bike ride in the park or a dance class or ice skating. It will be whatever is appropriate to you. We will cover this in full later.

It is worth mentioning here how we, as individuals, sabotage our chances of success by limiting our beliefs. For example, how often do we say 'I cannot do .....' or 'I won't be able to.....' or 'I don't have the ..... to do it'?

These are called limiting beliefs and I will show you how to overcome these. You can then use this in every area of your life.

In relation to exercise, I often hear people say 'Oh, I can't exercise' or 'I don't like exercise' and the like. These are all excuses because we exercise every day all day. Getting up, sitting down, walking to the fridge etc are all exercising. We have to decide what exercise we like and what we don't like. Would you like to dance with your partner or spend an hour in the gym?

You do not have to do anything you really don't want to. When I talk later about exercise, just keep in mind that exercise is only using our body's natural movements to physically achieve something we want.

Eat Less or Exercise More

Doing this in the right proportions can certainly get you to your objectives quickly and easily. But you must balance this so that you can achieve this day after day for the rest of your life.

Remember, this is all about you having fun, being less stressed, looking and feeling how you want to. It is about how you want to run your life for you. It is not about sacrifice or deprivation. It is not about pain, sweat and tears.

Balance is the key. I will help you create a balance that you can take forward as a part of you forever.

Some people say that they cannot eat less and that means they must exercise more. Others say that they cannot exercise so they must eat less.

I don't believe either of them.

Your beliefs are the key to every process you follow. They are the key to every strategy you use to get what you want.

Some people believe they can and some believe they can't. I know that they both can.

In the planning section of the book we will look at the balance needed between eating less and exercising more.

Eating better food

Eating fresh, well prepared, healthy food is obviously better for us than the pre-prepared, high salt content; high sugar convenience foods the big companies want us to buy.

But for some of us, we cannot afford organic food or the time to shop separately for each item. We have to shop at supermarkets and have to take what they offer that is within our budget.

By shopping carefully at a supermarket and by knowing which foods our bodies' processes easily, we can help greatly our enjoyment of what we eat and our weight management.

I should mention here that we will be covering toxins in detail in chapter 7. Toxins are not necessarily bad foods. They are foods that our bodies do not digest or deal with very well. They have a detrimental effect on our energy systems. We call them Individual Energy Toxins (IETs). They are probably the single most important contributory factor in poor energy.

Understanding them is critical in a successful long-term weight management system. IETs are different for different people, hence the name "individual". The most common toxins are wheat, corn, dairy, eggs and soy. For example, I am highly affected by wheat which reduces my energy levels dramatically whereas it has no effect on my wife. Coffee has no detrimental effect on me but upsets her energy systems. So it is horses for courses.

I believe that it is better to eat less of a healthy food than loads of an unhealthy food. I also believe that it is more enjoyable and more satisfying to eat something that actually tastes good. When you reduce your toxin levels, your body's natural systems take over and you will start to want different foods. Instead of reaching for the chocolate you might reach for the fruit and **want to** reach for the fruit. If this seems a bit far fetched, it isn't, it has happened to many a chocoholic and they cannot believe it.

Toxins can be your washing powder, perfume and other things you inhale. A reduction in toxin intake will significantly improve your energy levels. I will show you how to test for toxins in your system.

It's all in the mind – or is it?

Over-eating, under-eating and the various other 'eating' issues we face everyday have a lot to do with the mind. I will explain how certain aspects of the mind works as we progress.

By understanding why the mind guides us to do things we do not necessarily want to do and why we develop habits; we can learn to control both the conscious and unconscious parts. Then we will be in total control and any decision we make in relation to our weight management will be 100% ours.

As I have identified earlier, there are at least 10 reasons why we eat. Two are great reasons and the other eight or more revolve around some form of anxiety whether this is addictive behaviour or habit based.

I will teach you how to eliminate all but the two great reasons and thereby liberate you to really enjoy your food. By the way, most thin people do naturally what I will show you.

What's right for you?

At all stages of this programme you must do what you know is right for you. However, if what I ask does not offend your religious or other deeply held beliefs or your values system, then PLEASE do as I ask for the first 12 days.

After this, it is up to you. Do whatever is right for you. But remember, if you want to control your weight and you are committed to it, my programme really works if you follow it for the majority of the time.

Chapter 6
Realistic objectives and measurements

Ever set a target you could never reach even if you were Superman or Wonderwoman? Yes? We all have and what a waste they are- aren't they!

We will now set targets that we know we can reach. Not daft ones like losing 1lb in 2 years, or 10 pounds in a day but something reasonable.

If your objective is to lose weight initially to a level you can control and be happy at then I would like you to set a maximum target of 2lb (1kg) a week for the first 12 weeks.

Preferably less if you can. An ideal target is 1lb (500g) a week. This will provide you with a very achievable target and you will hardly notice any change in your normal lifestyle to achieve this. At this rate you would lose 52 lbs in a year or 3 stone 10 lbs (23.6 kg).

Below, write in your targets. Reaching a target creates great feelings of achievement. So I would rather you set 1lb a week and achieved 1.2 lb a week than set 2 lb a week and achieved 1.5 lb. I know you would have missed out on 0.3 lb that week but it's not all about weight. It's also about feeling good and feeling in control.

How much (1kg = 2.2lb)

Lb
Kg

By when

(weeks)

What you will look like (describe you)

What you will feel like (describe it)

What will you hear from others and in your thoughts (describe it)

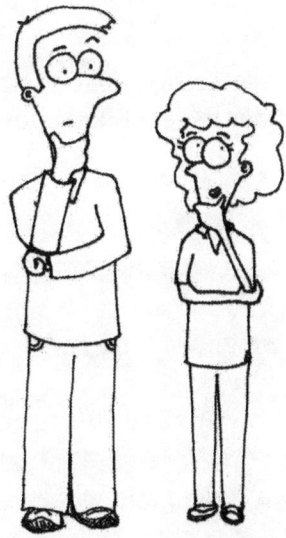

How we will measure success

Lb (or Kg)/12 days

Lb (or Kg)/12 weeks

Review so far

Believe it or not, we have come most of the way already to you controlling your weight at the level you choose. Already...........

o   We know why we eat

o   We know why we eat when we are not hungry

o   We know about weight management

o   We know about how anxiety affects our eating habits

o   We know what we can do and what doesn't work

o   We know what we want to achieve

o   We know how we will measure our success

o   We are committed to achieving it

So we are ready to get on witwh learning how we are going to do it. Sorry to disappoint you but you already know. You may not know that you know – but you do. I will show you how. So be prepared for the 'Uh Huh' moments and the 'I know that....' moments.

We are now ready to design your individual weight management system specifically for you. Firstly, before we do, you need to know about and understand the basic techniques we will use that form part of the success system. These are Thought Field Therapy (TFT) which we will use to eliminate addictive urges, anxiety, fear and cravings and secondly Individual Energy Toxins which we will learn how to identify and use to give our bodies the best chance of success.

Chapter 7
Thought Field Therapy (TFT)

TFT or to give it its full title, Callahan Techniques® Thought Field Therapy® was created and developed by Dr Roger Callahan. TFT is the simple, easy to use and effective way in which we will eliminate the anxieties, fears and stresses about weight management.

Often described as the power therapy for the 21st century, TFT is an 'Accredited Therapy' by the National Health Service Trust Association and, if you are in the UK, can be offered by your local Doctor as a referral to a TFT practitioner for all forms of personal, physical and emotional issues.

TFT uses tapping on your energy meridians to put your body's systems in a state where they can work at their most effective and efficient.

The basic things you need to know about TFT are as follows (we will be repeating things as we progress so you do not need to commit these to memory):

•   Thought Field.

    When we think of anything, that thought is formed in a thought field for the time we are thinking about it. A similar concept to a magnetic field or gravitational field, it exists whilst we are in it. For TFT to work, you must be in the thought field. For example, a craving treatment will not work if you are not thinking about the craving.

- Perturbation in the Thought Field.

  Perturbation is defined as a cause of mental disquietude. It is something that upsets the thought field and brings with it unwanted negative emotional upset.

- PR.

  This is an effect known as Psychological Reversal. Psychological Reversal (PR) is literally a state of reversed electrical polarity in the body. This state or condition blocks natural healing and prevents otherwise effective treatments from working. I will show you how to correct it.

- Individual Energy Toxins (IET).

  These are any foods that, after eating them, you feel bloated, unwell, sluggish, or your heart rate rises or you get any form of uncomfortable feeling. They are foods that reduce your energy and your body's defense capability. We will learn basic techniques for identifying your Individual Energy Toxins.

- Tapping points.

  These are areas on the body where I will be asking you to use two fingers to tap. When I do, please tap firmly enough to put some energy into the tapping spot but not hard enough to hurt you. The sequence of tapping and process will be explained as we need them.

- Algorithm.

  An algorithm is simply a strictly defined sequence of tapping that is effective in eliminating a particular issue. For example, the algorithm for anxiety is different to the algorithm for cravings. Treat an algorithm like a combination lock. In the right order of numbers the lock will open. In the wrong order it will not.

For the rest of this part of the programme please just do as I ask without question or analysis. This way the system will work best for you and it will all become clear as we progress. Nothing that I will ask you to do is invasive nor will it do you any harm whatsoever.

However, I want you to know about TFT in depth and we are very fortunate to have, in Appendix 1, an introduction to TFT, written by its creator, Dr Roger Callahan. This will help you to understand fully its power and how it can help you in every area of your life and not only weight management.

TFT uses tapping on defined spots on the body's energy meridians to collapse the perturbations in the thought field and, thereby, eliminate the emotional upset whether this is a craving, anxiety, fear or phobia etc.

TFT is very powerful, rapid and totally safe therapy. My only word of warning is to be prepared to be amazed. It is so quick it can leave a state of confusion when an old issue disappears so quickly. Do not be concerned about this as it is a totally normal reaction.

Before we start any TFT process we **must** think of the issue we want to eliminate (we call this tuning the thought field).

We then identify on a scale of 1 to 10 how upsetting or distressing this thought makes us feel. A measure of 1 would be no distress and a measure of 10 would be the worst possible. We call this the Subjective Unit of Distress (SUD) and we will use this to measure our success after the TFT treatment. While the 1 to 10-point scale is the most common self-report, *any* scale or description of graduated intensity is acceptable, as long as you are able to be consistent in measuring it.

It is also important to emphasize you should come up with the number that best represents the degree of upset at this moment just thinking about the problem, ***not*** how you have felt in the past or how you anticipate you might feel in the future.

We then make sure that we are not Psychologically Reversed (PR). We do this by tapping 15 times on the side of our hand. We tap the karate chop part of the side of the hand (the fleshy bit).

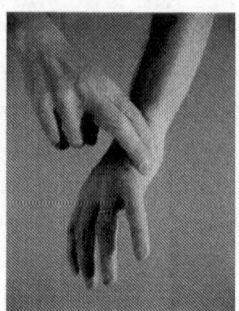

We then carry out the tapping sequences (explained below).

We then take a SUD reading and measure how far we have reduced the upset.

We continue the process described below until the issue is eliminated.

In summary,

- You have taken a SUD (1 – 10) for the condition
- You have made sure you have cleared any PR (psychological reversal)
- You have your sequence of points to tap.
- You must tap these points in the exact sequence given.
- You must tap each point at least 15 times.
- You must tap hard enough to put energy in but not had enough to hurt
- We take another SUD (1 – 10)
- We continue until the issue is eliminated (SUD at 1 or 2)

Please note that you can tap with either hand on either side of the body e.g. under your right eye or left eye as the energy meridians are symmetrical around the body.

How a TFT tapping sequence is applied.

The Components of some selected TFT Algorithms and the tapping sequences

Algorithms follow a standard well-defined pattern. By completing each step strictly in the order that they are prescribed, you will be performing effective TFT in the most efficient manner possible. There is one standard protocol for all Algorithms, and it conforms to the architecture commonly present in TFT. The places we will ask you to tap are shown in the following diagram

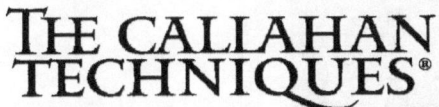

THE CALLAHAN TECHNIQUES®

Treatment Points
© 1994 Roger J. Callahan

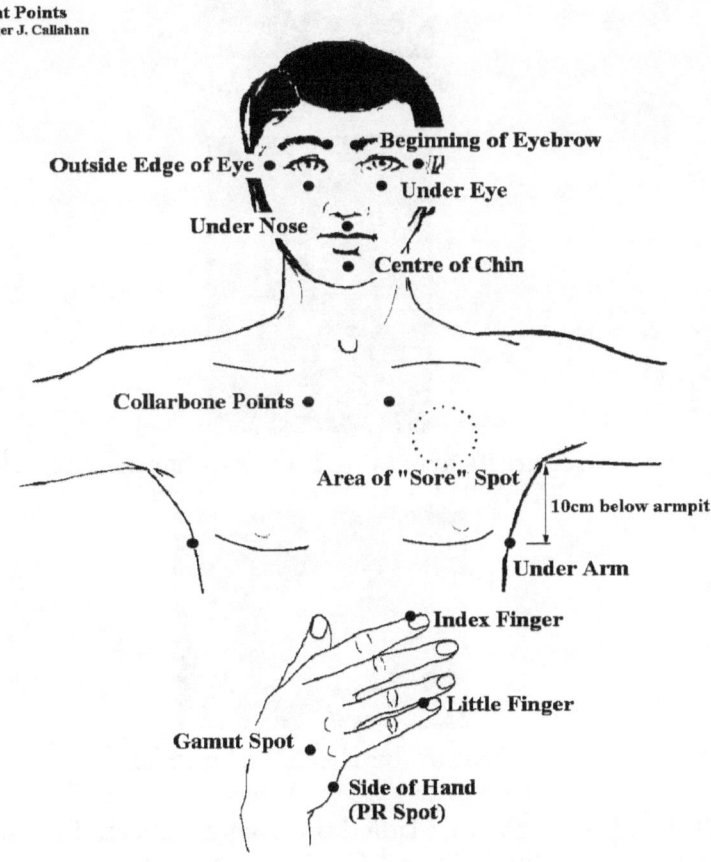

Beginning of Eyebrow

Outside Edge of Eye

Under Eye

Under Nose

Centre of Chin

Collarbone Points

Area of "Sore" Spot

10cm below armpit

Under Arm

Index Finger

Little Finger

Gamut Spot

Side of Hand
(PR Spot)

To illustrate this, the TFT protocol for the treatment of anxiety (this is the one we will use most) is shown below:

In an abbreviated form, it can be written: **e, a, c, 9g, sq**.

In TFT terminology this means

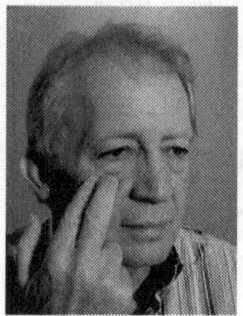

Under the eye (e)

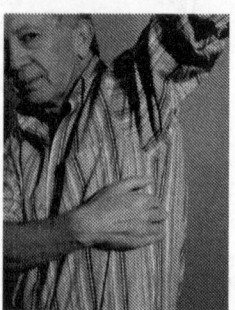

Under the arm (a) (4 inches under armpit)

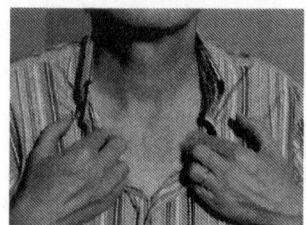

Just under the collarbone (c)

The sequence above is called the 'Majors'. A set of majors can be 1 tapping point or many

After the majors we carry out the 9 gamut treatments (9g) (detailed below)

This is a number of treatments in one sequence that we always use with every algorithm. It works by continuously tapping the Gamut Spot all the way through the sequence (allowing a minimum of about 10 taps for each step).

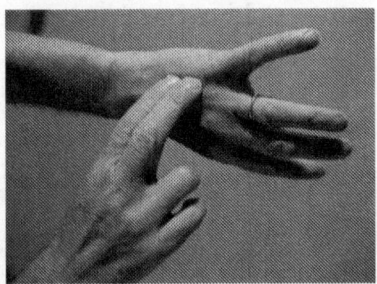

Gamut Spot

The gamut Spot is located between the knuckles of the tiny finger and ring finger and, in the valley between them 1 inch towards your wrist.

Now carry out the following (you are allowed to laugh while doing this):

Tap the Gamut spot continually throughout this sequence.

1. Close your eyes
2. Open your eyes
3. Move your eyes down and to one side
4. Move your eyes down and to the other side
5. Roll the eyes in a circle in one direction
6. Roll the eyes in a circle in the opposite direction
7. Hum a tune out loud for about 5 seconds
8. Count out loud from one to five
9. Hum the tune again aloud for about 5 seconds

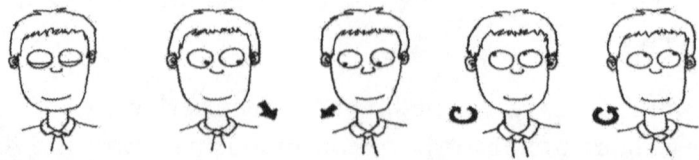

Now practice the 9g treatment until you can do it without the notes. It will come quite quickly after one or two practices.

After the 9g treatment we repeat the majors. This is represented by the term 'SQ' in the algorithm

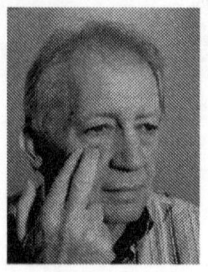
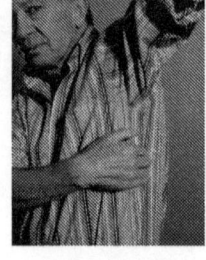
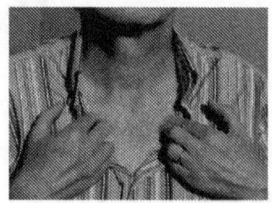

Under eye (e)   Under Arm (a)   Collarbone (c)

We will cover all the abbreviations later. The complete treatment sequence is known as a **Holon**. Each Holon is a "**9 gamut sandwich,**" including:

Majors (top slice), 9g (sandwich filling) and Majors (bottom slice).

Each TFT sequence is different for different solutions. It can contain 1 major or 6 majors or anywhere in between.

Now practice the majors above.

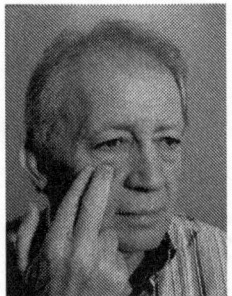

Under the eye (e)

Locate the fleshy part under the eye socket and tap about 15 times.

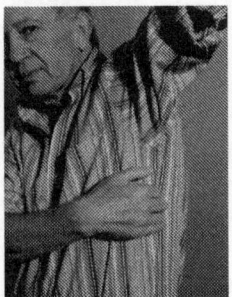

Under the arm (a) (4 inches under armpit)
Then locate the under arm spot and tap 15 times.

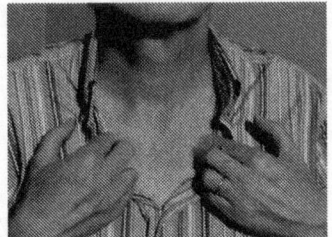

Just under the collarbone (c)
Then locate the collarbone point and tap 15 times.

Tap hard enough to put energy into the body but not hard enough to cause you pain. Simple? How do you feel now even without having thought of a problem?

Repeat this sequence (e, a, c) until you are used to it without referring to the notes or pictures.

If you are concerned about locating the collarbone spot, you have an inch or two leeway either side. However, for accuracy follow your windpipe down to the **V** notch where your collarbones meet your sternum. At the bottom of the notch move an inch down and an inch across to the fleshy part just under the collarbone. This is the collarbone spot.

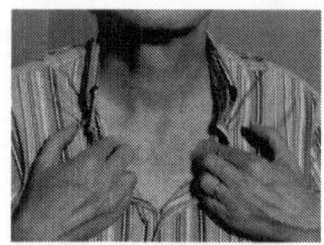

Now practice the 9 Gamut treatments.

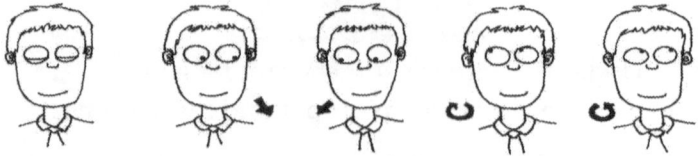

In a treatment sequence we have majors, 9G, majors. This would look like

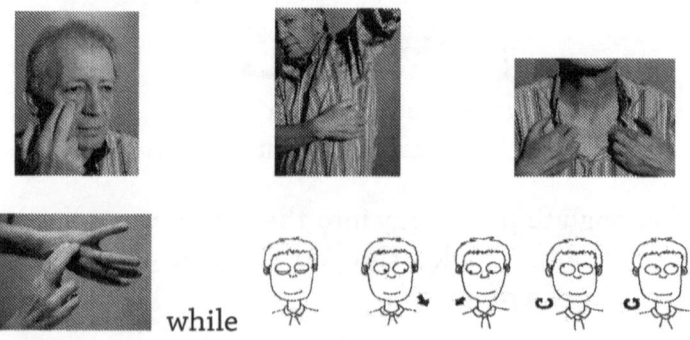

while

Hum of 5 seconds – count 1 to 5 – hum for 5 seconds

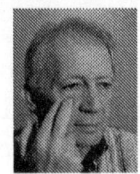 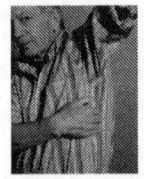 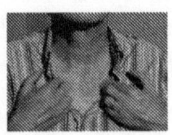

In a treatment sequence, when your SUD has reached a level of 2 or less I suggest that you complete the floor to ceiling eye roll.

The floor to ceiling eye roll should be used at the end of all of the Algorithm treatments when the SUD is a 2 or lower. It will usually bring a SUD of 2 to a 1. If not, go back to where you were in the Protocol and do the next step.

To complete an effective floor to ceiling eye roll, stand or sit upright, hold the head level, move the eyes (not the head) down to the floor. Tap the Gamut spot continuously while you slowly raise the eyes to the ceiling (about 10 seconds for the complete sequence).

This treatment can also be done by itself for the purposes of stress reduction or rapid relaxation.

Just before we finish the technical stuff I want to cover Psychological Reversal (PR) in more detail and explain something about Individual Energy Toxins (IET). Both of these topics can help greatly in every part of your life and not just weight management.

Psychological Reversals and their Correction - The TFT Law of Reversal

Psychological Reversal (PR) is literally a state of reversed polarity in the body.

This state or condition blocks natural healing and prevents otherwise effective treatments from working. Dr Callahan discovered that a person who is in a state of psychological reversal is unable to respond to an otherwise effective TFT treatment or any other effective treatment.

A person can be psychologically reversed in just one, a select few, or many areas of life. For instance, a person who has a "mental block" against learning mathematics might be psychologically reversed only in that area and not with other subjects.

How to Recognize a Psychological Reversal (PR)

- TFT or other treatments (e.g. a medical treatment that is normally effective) do not work
- Reversing words, concepts, and / or numbers
- Grumpy, irritable, negative mood
- Self-sabotaging behaviour
- Negative self-talk
- Procrastination
- Having a "mental block" in a particular area, such as mathematics, writing, computers, etc

Once PR has been corrected, which is an extraordinarily simple process, approximately 80% of people who did not respond to a TFT treatment will report the expected decrease in SUD after they repeat the same treatment.

Psychological Reversal Corrections

At any level, once PR has been corrected, begin the TFT treatment again from the beginning.

Correction for PR

Indication: *Little or no change in SUD after the majors*

Tap the Specific PR spot on the side of the hand (karate chop point) about 15 times while focusing on the problem.

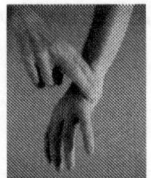

PR Spot
Side of Hand (Karate Chop Point)

Repeat the majors. Check SUD. If SUD has not dropped 2 or more points, go to Recurring PR (Appendix 1).

There are a number of other treatments for PR but for normal purposes, tapping the side of the hand (Karate Chop point) is usually sufficient.

What is an Individual Energy Toxin?

The identification of Individual Energy Toxins (IETs) and their elimination will take you well over half way to achieving your weight management objectives. Therefore, it is extremely important that you read this section over and over until you understand it. More explanation is given on Dr Roger Callahan's website at www.tftrx. com

Please remember that we are talking about things that are toxins specifically to you. They are not 'toxic' components in the wider sense. For example, wheat is a toxin for me but not for my wife. This does not make wheat a bad product. It makes it inadvisable for me. These reactions are unique to individuals and affect these energy systems in a specific way. Therefore they are called Individual Energy Toxins (IETs).

It is important to minimize the level of toxins in your system as a high level can cause PR and affect the effectiveness of the TFT treatment.

IET substances may be found in everyday life situations and are harmless to most individuals. For some individuals, however, these substances can cause serious problems.

Practitioners trained in TFT Diagnosis or higher can identify IETs for you.

For the weight loss programme, we will teach you some basic methods of identification and treatment. For more advanced work and to see a really fantastic effect on your energy levels and positive outlook on life, you can use the services of a TFT specialist or you can buy a kit from Callahan Techniques www.tftrx.com , developed by Dr Roger Callahan, called "Sensitivities, Intolerances, and TOXINS: How to Identify and Neutralize Them with TFT." These substances can be ingested, inhaled, or contacted.

Some IETs might be expected, e.g., tobacco, pesticides, and various organic chemicals (in clothing, carpets, upholstery, paint, etc.); however, some of the most common IETs are unexpected, e.g., wheat, corn, eggs, milk and other dairy products, perfumes, laundry soap or detergents, scented tissue, shampoo, toothpaste or deodorants.

The Barrel Effect

The barrel effect is an important factor in understanding toxins. Dr. Doris Rapp explained this very concisely in her video, *Environmentally Sick Schools*. The body deals with each suspect food, or other toxin, as if it were being contained in a barrel where it can be isolated before being disposed of. One toxin may not necessarily become a problem; however, if the barrel is filled to overflowing, then a problem can develop.

The toxin spills over to exert a physiological or psychological effect on the body.

An interesting question is this—when someone "clears" a toxin, is he/she increasing the barrel size or actually removing the item from a list of potentially harmful items?

The direct evidence of our standard approach in TFT suggests that we can indeed strengthen an individual (i.e., increase the size of the toxin barrel) with our treatments. We can eliminate problems, even though the person's problem might originate in toxin exposure.

Dr. Arthur Coca (1994), in *The Pulse Test*, maintained that we do not become allergic by over-indulging in a particular substance. Instead, our allergens are determined by our heredity. In other words, he suggested that the barrel for some foods will never overflow unless that food was an inherited allergen.

Indicators of Toxic Sensitivity

- Malaise
- Water Retention
- Fidgeting/Restless Feet
- Hyperactivity/Labile Emotions
- Constipation/Diarrhoea (on their own or alternating)
- Red Ears/Blotchy Skin (neurodermatitis)
- Sticky Faeces
- Fatigue after meals
- Panic Attacks
- Hyperactivity
- Insomnia
- Irritability
- Obesity
- Bloatedness
- Nausea
- Cravings (e.g. for specific foods)

From the above you can see the effect on the body that IETs have. They also stop the body operating effectively and add seriously to weight issues.

Can IETs be "cleared"?

We are often asked if an IET itself can be treated with TFT (or some other method) so that the person can continue to consume the identified substance without ill effects. Given that toxins can often be favourite foods, we all wish that this were so!

Myself and other Callahan Techniques® approved advanced TFT practitioners have experimented extensively with several so-called "toxin clearing" treatments and are aware of the extensive claims that are being made for a number of such methods. It has been our experience that these methods **do not** neutralize an IET to the point where a person can continue to consume a substance without the ill effects.

This can be extremely dangerous because some ill effects have *no apparent symptoms*, and the person incorrectly believes that the toxin has been "cleared." In fact, the toxin has not been cleared, and the person risks his/her health without even knowing it. This may only reveal itself when the person has become very ill, often too late for resolution to take place.

Since an IET can often be a person's favourite foods (i.e., they have become addicted to the IET), they desperately want to believe that the toxicity can be "cleared" so they can continue to indulge. Hence, they can become susceptible to the false claims of those who say that they can clear toxins.

Once your problem has been eliminated you should continue to avoid toxins for at least two months while you are totally symptom free. After that you should re-introduce them with care. Contact your therapist or trainer at once if the symptoms return.

In the case of toxins that cannot be avoided, consult a practitioner trained in TFT Voice Technology or TFT Diagnosis who has taken the Advanced TFT training.

I will show you here some simple ways to identify and clear a toxin. Clearing toxins is covered in depth at the 1-day weight control training course based on this book.

The Pulse Test

Arthur F. Coca, MD was a top allergist who founded the medical organization of allergists and edited the major journal. He was a Professor at Columbia University and was highly regarded in his profession until his discovery of the role of the pulse in identifying allergens. This simple test caused him to be ostracized.

Mrs. Coca was a medical researcher. She was hospitalized with angina and given only five years to live. Mrs. Coca was given a morphine derivative while in hospital, and her pulse began beating so fast that it could not be counted easily–faster than 180 beats per minute. Mrs. Coca mentioned that her pulse often raced after certain meals. This led to Dr. Coca to explore and find that the pulse increases with the ingestion of an allergen/toxin. He suggested that she count her pulse following the intake of SINGLE FOODS to see if other culprits might be identified.

He was able to experiment with many of his patients and to develop a simple and efficient means of identifying the substances, which affected the health of his patients. His small and readable book, *The Pulse Test*, is highly recommended for a full explanation of his theories and techniques. *The Pulse Test* provides extensive background information and instruction for using this method.

The base method is:

- Find a baseline pulse (your normal pulse rate sitting and standing. Add together and halve), and compare this with the pulse immediately after exposure to a potential toxin and up to an hour later.
- A resting heart rate of more than 84 beats per minute usually indicates that the person has been exposed to an IET.

- An increase in pulse rate of more than a few beats per minute after exposure to a toxin will also indicate sensitivity.
- A difference of over 10 beats per minute between sitting and standing will indicate the presence of a toxin.

Proximity Toxins

Once you have carried out the corrections for PR i.e. Side of Hand 15 times and/or under the nose 15 times and you still have difficulty reducing your SUD, it may be due to a proximity toxin. The following treatment can be applied after the reversal treatment for PR2 (under the nose) and before Collarbone Breathing (CB2). See the previous diagram for the exact points to tap.

Environmental Toxin Correction
Tap the Index Finger 15 times.
Tap the Specific PR spot (side of hand) 15 times.
Then, repeat the treatment that hadn't previously worked.

Take a look at Dr Callahan's Introduction to TFT in Appendix 1 for a more detailed explanation on IETs.

Keep a list of foods you eat and any adverse symptoms that arise from eating them. Check them for being an IET and log down those you should avoid. A prepared log sheet and instructions on identifying toxins can be obtained by emailing us at info@oh-crikey.com

That is the end of the technical stuff. I trust you found it simple to follow. If you have any concerns about it, go back and read it again and practice the sequences until you feel comfortable with them.

It is now time to use what we have learned and practice some real TFT.

TFT Algorithms for anxiety and cravings

To remind us, an algorithm is a recipe of one or more points which together comprise a treatment that has been found to work for a particular problem (such as anxiety or stress) in approximately 70% to 90% percent of cases.

The algorithms you will be using most are:

E, a, c, 9g, sq for anxiety and stress, and (comic strip)
C, e, c, 9g, sq for addictive urge (comic strip)

In the above example for anxiety this would mean in longhand - E, a, c, 9g, e, a, c.

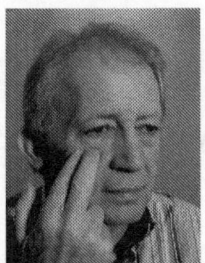

Under eye 15 times (e)

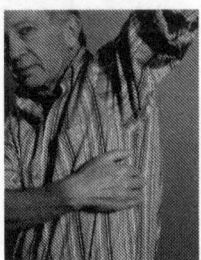

Under arm 15 times (a)

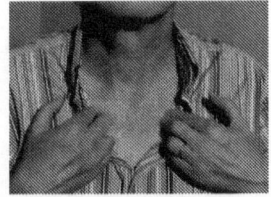

Collarbone 15 times (c)

Steve McNulty

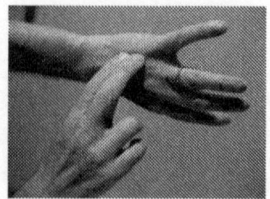

Gamut Spot tap continually (G)

Close eyes
Open Eyes
Eyes down right
Eyes down left
Roll eyes in circle right
Roll eyes in circle left

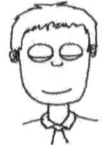 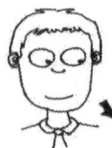 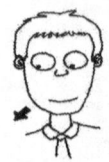 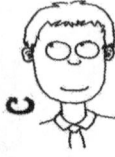 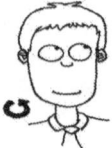

Hum out loud for 5 seconds
Count 1 to 5 out loud
Hum out loud for 5 seconds
47

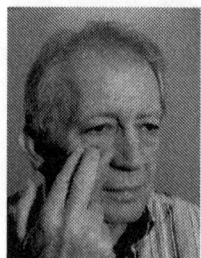

Under eye 15 times (e)

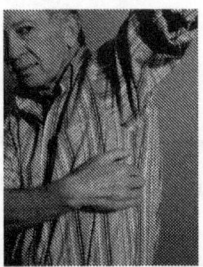

Under arm 15 times (a)

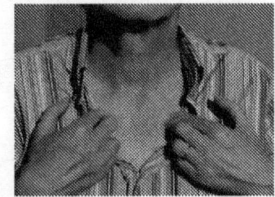

Collarbone 15 times (c)

If your SUD is 2 or less now carry out the floor to ceiling eye roll.

Now practice these until you can do it without the notes. It won't take long.

Once you have mastered the technique, you can use it to clear any anxiety, craving or fear you have. The complete process becomes:

- Clear any PR (15 taps on the Side of hand point)

- Think of the issue (tune the thought field)

- Establish a SUD (rate on a scale of 1 – 10 how bad it is)

- Correct for PR (tap the side of your hand 15 times (karate chop point))

- While thinking of the issue

- Carry out the algorithm MAJORS

- o If your SUD has dropped by 2 or more
  - Carry out the 9G sequence followed by the MAJORS

- o If your SUD has not dropped by 2 or more
  - Tap the majors again until it does

- o If your SUD doesn't drop, correct for PR and/or Toxins

- After completing the 9G repeat the MAJORS

- Go around this process until the SUD is 2 or less

- Carry out the floor to ceiling EYE ROLL

If after all this you cannot get the SUD to drop, use the alternative algorithms in Appendix 3.

Now you have a simple and easy technique to help you overcome cravings and negative thoughts. You can also this and the techniques I show you later on for how to break old bad habits and create good new ones.

That is a brief introduction to the technique I am using. When you are comfortable with this and want to know more, Roger's introduction to TFT can be found in Appendix 1

Let us recap.......

- We know why we eat
- We know why we eat when we are not hungry
- We know about how anxiety affects our eating habits
- We know about weight management
- We know what we can do to control our weight and what doesn't work
- We know what we want to achieve and when
- We know how we will measure our success
- We are committed to achieving our objectives
- We have learned about Energy Meridian Systems

- We have learned about Thought Field Therapy ® and how Anxiety is the root cause of the majority of distress.
- We have learned about PR and how to reverse it
- We now know about Individual Energy Toxins (IETs), how important they are to us (to eliminate them), how to identify and treat them
- We have learned how to self-administer TFT algorithm treatments to eliminate the anxiety and urges that are the cause of eating when we are not hungry

You now have all the elements needed to understand how we can manage our weight at the level we choose. We now need to put it all together into your own weight management system.

Chapter 8
The success plan

Following my success programme will give you...

The benefits

- You will get control back in your life
- You will decide what you do and what you don't do
- You will set your own targets and achieve them

The drawbacks

- You will have no excuses

How you will look

- How you want to

How you will feel

- Great
- Proud of yourself

Please bear in mind as you read on that I will be showing you over 30 ways to help you successfully manage your weight. I will then summarise these into 4 sets of 6 easy steps based on eating, exercise, the mind and others. I will ask you to complete as many as you can for the first 12 days and then you can relax and decide on any 12 from the first 18 and as many of the final 6 as you feel are appropriate for you. This will give you total flexibility and allow you to design the system that suits your lifestyle and your preferences.

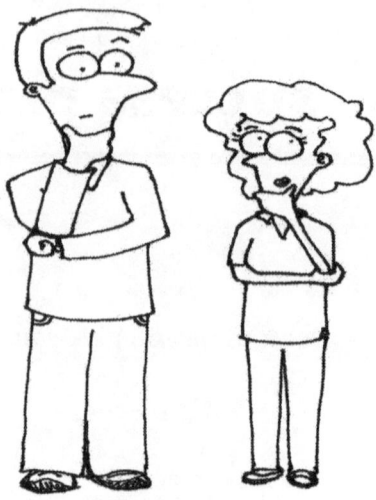

How you can help yourself everyday and do nothing else I ask

If you do nothing else, please follow the basic guidelines below. If you do, you will start to get control of your weight and then you will be able to begin to manage it.

Doing the things below will help but for making a real difference you need to do as I ask for the first 12 days and then as I ask for the remainder of the first 12 weeks.

I know we are repeating things – but they are important.

Commit to do some, preferably all, of the following from NOW.

Check yourself for IETs

Make a list with two sides, one side for toxins and one for food that is OK. It is equally important to note down the food that is OK and this will become the bigger list very quickly.

Read food labels when shopping and avoid any item that contains one of your toxins.

Avoid IETs at all costs

Correct yourself for PR regularly throughout the day by tapping the side of your hand (Karate Chop Point) 15-20 times in quick succession.

Walk places

Exercise doesn't mean the gym, sweating on a treadmill, being out of breath, leotards and the like. It means moving your body more than you do now.

Choose places to go and things to do where you can walk.

Park further away from the entrance at the supermarket or work and walk.

Go for a short stroll when you have 5 minutes spare.

If you have never walked anywhere start by walking anywhere for 1 minute on day one and add 1 minute a day until on day twelve you will be walking for 12 minutes a day.

Shop only on a full stomach

Go shopping after you have eaten a meal. Don't go shopping when you feel you are hungry – please.

With everything you eat – eat it slowly

We all remember being told as kids to chew our food properly. We only did if we were being watched. There wasn't enough time to eat when there was far more interesting and important things to do – like play with our friends.

Well, Mother was right again. I hate to admit it but this is one "old wives' tale" that is true and is really important.

We tend to hoover our food into our digestive system and thereby give it no chance of working properly. Have you noticed how we nearly always have the next mouthful of food ready and poised in front of our mouth before we have even started to swallow the last one? We seem more interested in what is going to go into our mouths than what is in there already.

Everyone is in a rush these days and so we have forgotten how to eat properly. Slow down and enjoy your food.

Take this opportunity to change this around. Do not start to get the next mouthful ready until you have finished what is in your mouth now.

Put your knife and fork down between mouthfuls. Savour the taste of every mouthful of food.

Re-learn how food tastes and the texture of good food. How tastes combine to provide a pleasurable eating experience.

Have you ever wondered how we got to know that mint sauce was good with lamb? How cranberries fit with turkey. Cinnamon with apple etc. We have to be able to taste our food to appreciate this. To taste we need to chew. Chewing requires us to take our time.

Try it – you will be surprised what you normally eat really tastes like.

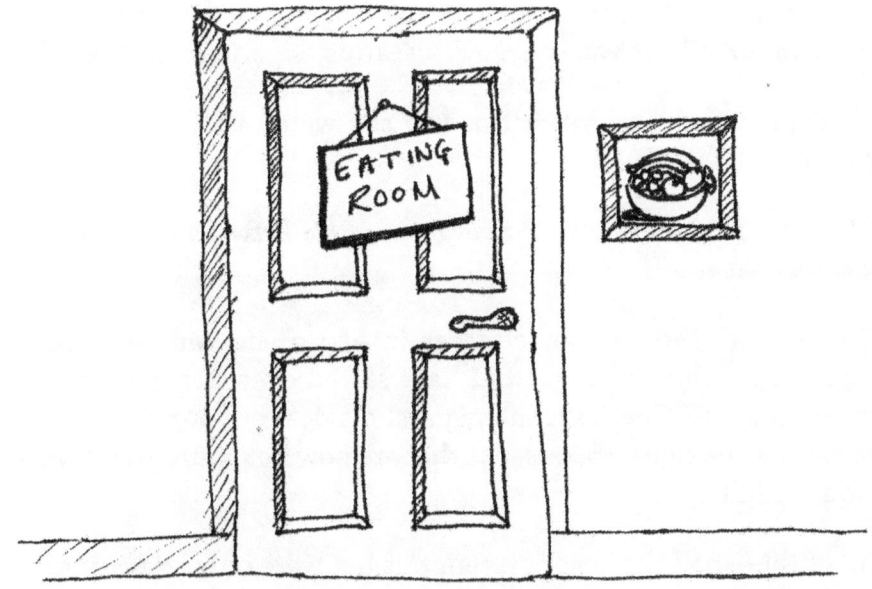

Have only one place in the house to eat (the Eating Room)

This should be a room, say the Dining Room, where there is no TV, no Radio, no music, just a place for eating.

I want you to eat only in the 'Eating Room'.

For example, you are sitting in the lounge in front of your favourite TV programme and your partner offers you a cup of tea. You accept and they also offer you a biscuit or a bowl of nibbly things. I would like you to say no to these. We know that this is difficult.

So you are allowed to say yes but you must have had a drink, you must be hungry and you must eat them in the 'eating' room with no TV, radio, music or any other distraction.

If you are distracted when you eat, you do not taste the food, you do not enjoy the food and you do not realise how much you are eating. You do not realise when you are full.

Taking away all distractions (other than conversation with a companion) allows you to enjoy the eating experience to the full.

No deprivation, you can eat or you can watch the TV – it's your choice.

When the food doesn't taste that great decide between the waste bin and your waste bin

"Think of all the starving children in Africa", my Mother used to say to me. "Clean your plate. I have slaved over this and you are going to eat it". There are many psychological pressures put on us to eat, for the right reasons, but that are now not appropriate when we are adults.

All of these had the best of intentions but were only relevant to us as children. They have no relevance to us now as adults. If we eat it, or if we eat do not it, it still cannot go to the children in Africa!

You can decide where the waste goes. Does it go in the waste bin or in to your stomach as waste? It's your choice.

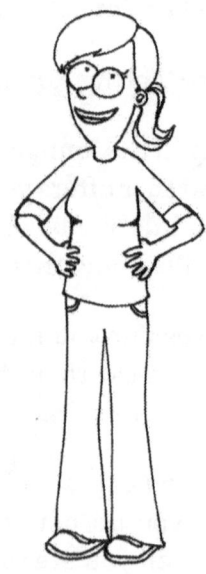

Feel proud of yourself

You have made a decision to take control of your weight. That means that you have made the decision to take control of your body and of your life.

Well done. You deserve to feel really proud of yourself.

Feel proud of yourself every time you say no to food when you are not hungry.

Feel proud of yourself when you realise that you have eaten a complete meal and tasted every mouthful.

Now let us look at how the mind works.

THE MIND MODEL

To understand fully why we have good and bad habits it helps to understand how the mind works.

Think of the Mind as being like an Iceberg. A small part of it is visible above the water. This is the conscious mind. The much larger part of it is below the water (unseen). This is the unconscious part.

The surface of the water (the barrier between the conscious mind and the unconscious mind is known as the Critical Faculty.

In our conscious mind we have all the day to day things like motivation and willpower. We have activities like logical thinking about how to do things. We evaluate our surroundings and take actions accordingly.

This is our conscious state. If you drive a car you will remember how, when you started, you had to consciously think about every thing you did. .Mirror, signal, manoeuvre. Clutch in, foot off throttle, change gear, clutch out, foot on throttle and so on.

After a while you started to do these things without conscious thought. You developed unconscious competence and developed a positive habit. You don't think about these things now – do you?

This is the same with any sport or pastime you enjoy. You started off thinking about everything you had to do. After many hours of practice things happen naturally and you can start to concentrate on developing your abilities further.

The only issue we have with willpower is that we have to remember to have it and use it. This requires us to have a permanent amount of constant motivation.

So the unconscious mind carries out many tasks for us all the time. Without it we would have difficulty in surviving.

Let's look at our bodily functions. For example breathing! Until I raised it here, when did you last think about having to breathe? We don't, because breathing is a bodily function looked after by our unconscious mind.

The unconscious mind stores our memories. Where? Who knows, but they are there and can be recalled by various means. Music is a powerful memory trigger.

We can recall feelings of happiness as children when we were given a treat for being good (normally chocolate).

The unconscious also triggers our emotions and feelings. Situations arise and we feel a certain way and our emotions come to the surface as upsets in our in our thoughts. In TFT we call this upset a "perturbation" in the thought field. We can allow this to happen or we can control them. This normally depends on how strong they are. My programme will help you control your feelings and emotions to create a more positive you. It will also allow you to eliminate the perturbations fully to release you from emotional upset.

The unconscious mind also holds our belief system formulated from years of experience and conditioning. These beliefs form the basis of our values and are one of the key elements to a successful weight management programme.

Beliefs can be changed in a split second. Yes they can. Have you ever had your belief in someone shattered by one negative comment from someone else? The same can happen about beliefs you hold related to you and to your weight.

The unconscious mind is great for developing habits and for making sure we re-enforce them at every possible opportunity. If we do something often enough the unconscious mind recognises the pattern and programmes it in to our 'habit' section. Then every time it is triggered the habit is re-enforced. For example, smoking after a meal is purely a habit.

Every habit we have is there because originally it provided us with a positive benefit. However, many of these were formed in childhood and the reasons are now not relevant and the habits need to be broken.

I will show you how to achieve this.

Our unconscious also provides all our protection mechanisms. It judges our flight or fight responses. It develops protection mechanisms for all sorts of potentially dangerous situations physically and psychologically. It always does the right thing based on our beliefs and habits.

You can create better, more advantageous ways, of providing this protection using my programme. This will give you great freedom and satisfaction.

The greatest benefit your unconscious gives you is your IMAGINATION.

Your mind does not normally distinguish between reality and any vividly imagined situation, without conscious intervention. If you have ever had a nightmare, you know how real it feels at the time.

You can use your imagination to do various things like making you feel good for absolutely no reason whatsoever.

You can use it to try out how to deal with something you have to face in the future.

If you can imagine yourself at the weight and shape you want, then, you can make it happen.

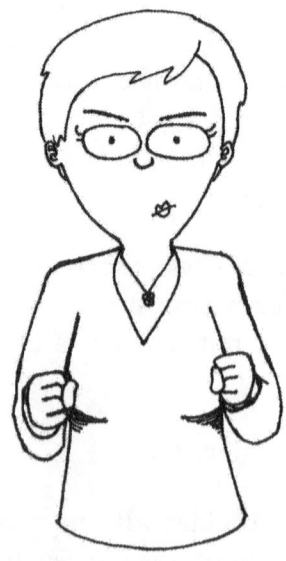

Willpower on its own isn't enough

As we said earlier, willpower requires you to remember to do something and when that is breaking a habit your unconscious can be stronger.

Imagination is key

Rather than rely on willpower, you will fire your imagination and let it re-establish your beliefs and habits to those you want to help you succeed.

Breaking unwanted habits is key

As a society, we have many old eating habits that are not relevant to how we live today. Some are:

- Finishing everything on your plate even if you are not hungry
- Having three square meals a day even when we are not hungry
- Standard eating times

Making good habits is key

You need to replace the old unnecessary habits with creative positive habits that help you and support you in managing your weight.

I will show you how to do this easily.

How to feel good for no reason at all

This is one of my favourite sections of the programme. I love feeling good for absolutely no reason whatsoever.

How do we do this? Well, you have done this in the past. When you get recall of a very happy event in your life and the memories flood back and you feel absolutely wonderful. It's as though you are there again enjoying the moment to the full.

That's all we are going to do here so just follow my instructions. Firstly read the next section through a few times and go through the process until you know it without the notes. It won't take long and it is really worth it.

I am going to ask you to visualize a time in the past or future. We can all visualize in our own way whether this is in pictures, sounds or feelings or all three. If you believe that you have difficulty in visualizing things, try this exercise.

Firstly, tap the side of your hand (SOH) 15 times and complete the following algorithm a, c, 9G, sq. That is, under arm, collarbone, 9 gamut, under arm, collarbone.

Then close your eyes and imagine being in your bathroom about to brush your teeth. Where is the brush and toothpaste, where are the taps in the sink, are you looking at yourself in the mirror? Whatever you saw, heard or felt then this is your way of visualizing. Some famous composers saw music in colours when they were composing. Some people only visualize in blurred images. It's OK. Do it your way.

For the first time you do this it is better to be sitting down in a quiet place where you have no distractions and can relax comfortably.

Are you sitting comfortably? Then we will begin.

Relax all the muscles in your body

Visualisation

Think of a time when you were really happy. The time when you were feeling really good. You know – that time! Careful.....

Take a few moments to do this while you concentrate on your breathing.

Once you have that time in your mind and you have the feeling of being there

Growing the feeling

Do you have a picture or an image? If you have a picture is it a still picture or a movie? If it is still then make it a movie. Make the picture or image bigger and keep making it bigger until it is life sized.

Are you in the image or looking at your self in the image? If you are looking at the image move into it so that you are part of it.

Make the colours brighter and bolder.

If you have a sound, make that sound fuller and louder and more energizing.

If you have a good feeling, make that feeling stronger and stronger.

Anchoring the feeling

Once you have the best feeling you have ever had, press your thumb and tiny finger together. Then relax

- Repeat this process five times. Then when you want to recall it just press your thumb and tiny finger together and bring the feeling back
- Recalling the feeling whenever you want

Now you have your good feeling anchor and you can recall those feelings whenever and wherever you want to. You can feel really good for no reason at all. Cool eh?

The more you practice this the stronger the anchor will become and the easier it will be to recall the good feelings whenever you need or want them.

Creating your support structure

Some people like to take on new techniques and methods on their own. They feel more in control that way and so, that is good for them.

If you, like me, need a support structure around you to help keep you focused and determined, then build one up very quickly.

At Oh-Crikey, I have provided a superb support structure for you and this is detailed at the end of the programme.

However, nothing is better than the love and support of your loved ones and those around you. So, tell them what you are doing. Ask for their encouragement and support. Ask for their patience with your new eating habits. Ask for their support in everything you do.

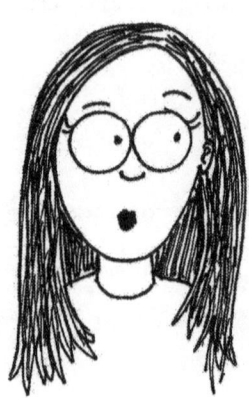

Chapter 9

The elements of the weight management system

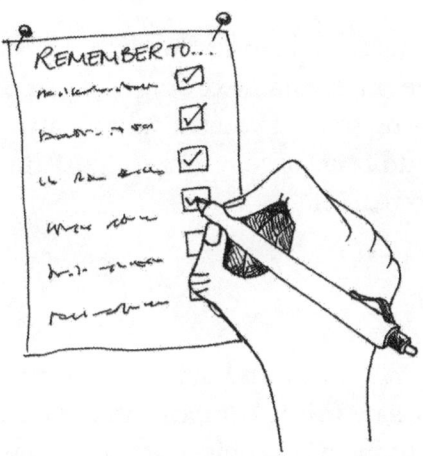

The 6 step easy way to eating management

Now we come to the big bit. The following key elements to managing your weight should be adhered to fully for the next 12 days, irrespective of anything.

Thirst

When you think you are hungry, drink as large a glass of water as you can.

Do this all the time. Carry a bottle of water with you everywhere for the first 12 weeks and when you think that you feel hungry, take a drink.

I prefer you to drink water. However, there has been much press lately stating that tea or coffee is OK as a substitute if you really would prefer to not drink water.

If caffeine is one of your toxins please avoid it as much as possible for the first 12 weeks.

If, after 10-15 minutes of having the drink of water, you are still hungry then move on to the next stage. If you are not hungry go off and do something to take your mind off eating, use the anxiety algorithm or the addictive urge/craving algorithm, use your anchor to feel good for no reason.

Eating

You have drunk your water and after 10-15 minutes you are still hungry. You **must** eat. This is compulsory for the first 12 days. You should always try to meet this objective. Once you have determined that you are really hungry you should not deprive your body of the fuel it needs, any longer than absolutely necessary.

Eat what your body tells you

Once you have passed the initial 12 week mark and you have identified your IETs and steered clear of them, you can eat what your body tells you to eat. By that time your tastes will have changed and you will desire food that tastes good and is good for you.

This is not the same as eating what you consciously think that you want. We want to eliminate food addictions and not strengthen them.

Until then I want you be sensible in what you eat. You must not go hungry. You must not feel bad about not eating something. Be sensible. Please check for toxins and avoid all food that can cause you any form of upset. Murphy's law will, of course, tell you that these will be all your favourite foods.

Later in the programme we will recall how you can stop any cravings. You already know how to feel good for no reason.

Being sensible and giving yourself a helping hand can mean, for example, having one less slice of bread or one less potato than normal or substituting another vegetable or more protein in its place.

Use a smaller plate than usual and put less on it. If you are still hungry after eating all that is on your plate and you are sure you are still hungry – put more on.

Eating is one of life's great pleasures. Enjoy it. Make a serious part of your daily life. Enjoy everything you eat.

Eat purposefully

Please, please, please chew your food fully. Put a moderate mouthful of food onto your fork or spoon and pop it into your mouth. Now put down your fork or spoon and chew your food. Chew for at least 25 times and preferably more if you can. Then swallow. Then get the next lot ready and start again.

Notice the tastes of the food. Notice the textures. Notice how you feel about this food having now chewed in thoroughly. Weird huh? Bizarre certainly.

After a few days of doing this you will begin to taste food properly again. You will enjoy your food more and you will be able to stop eating when you are full.

Stopping

As soon as you feel satisfied or you begin to feel full – STOP EATING. You don't need any more food. Your body is telling you this.

You do not have to clear your plate. You do not need to use your mouth as a waste bin instead of the proper waste bin.

You owe it to yourself to stop because you no longer need to eat. This also means you will be hungry earlier and so you get to eat nice food again sooner.

If you have cravings or urges, then tap them away with the algorithms you have learned or those in Appendix 3.

Don't waste good food. If you are not hungry, save your food and eat it later on when you are really hungry again.

Lapsing

It is OK to lapse occasionally. Lapses will slow down your progress but they will not stop it. You are not allowed to use lapses as an excuse for stopping controlling your weight.

If you do lapse, decide why you did it. Was the benefit worth the things you have lost?

Balance this against what you really want. Balance it against what is really important to you. Forgive yourself and get on with what is really important. Get in control of your weight.

If you know you have a big weekend coming up or a gastronomic holiday, plan to lapse and enjoy it. But please be sensible and still avoid IETs wherever possible.

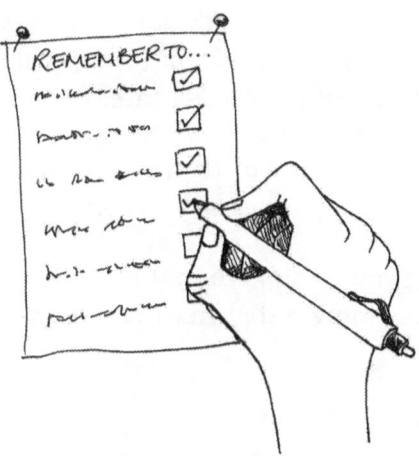

The 6 step easy way to exercise management

Some of us dread the word exercise and the images it conjures up. However, we exercise every day. We get up, walk around the house, do physical things etc. This is all exercise.

The following six easy steps to exercise management will help you to start to develop an exercise routine that will help you reach your objectives.

I would ask anyone who is about to take any additional exercise and has any reason to believe that this may not be appropriate for them to talk to their medical practitioner before embarking on an exercise regime.

As quickly or as slowly as suits you, I want to help you improve your heart rate. All the things I show you can be timed with a standard watch with a second hand.

Your heart rate is one of the keys to burning off fat or developing muscle or both. It is often a misconception that you need to 'work out' to burn off fat. This is not the case.

I will show you below how to work out your maximum heart rate and then how exercising at half of this (50%) will burn off fat faster than exercising at 80% of your heart rate.

But you don't need to do any of this. It will help and you will feel better but it is not strictly necessary to control your weight.

All I will be asking you to do is to build up over a 12 day period to walking 12 minutes more a day than you do now. After that it is up to you.

Walk places

Walk where and when you can and as often as you can.

When you park the car, park further away than normal from where you are going. Walk an extra hundred yards each time if you can.

Try to go out for a short walk everyday with your partner, dog, iPod, Walkman or yourself.

Start on Day 1 with a 1 minute walk. Add 1 minute a day for the next 11 days. On day 12 you will be walking for 12 minutes. Depending on how fast you walk this will be about or just over half a mile.

If you can find someone to walk with you can walk & talk together each day. You can ensure you both do it and you can help each other get the results you both want.

Do not put any strain on your body during this period. So, if you have a sprained knee, it is OK not to do this part of the programme – yet.

It is better to do a little often every week rather than a lot once a week.

Using the stairs

If and only if you are physically able to, use the stairs instead of the lift. For five stories in a building use the stairs for one and the lift for the other four or vice versa. Then, over time, build up to climbing to the second floor using the stairs, then the third floor. I suggest that you stop there and use the lift. Why, because it's a pain in the neck walking up more than 3 flights of stairs.

Laughing

Try getting a few videos or DVDs of comedy programmes you know will make you laugh out loud. Watch these as often as you can and enjoy a really good laugh.

Alternately, tune in to some of the comedy channels and laugh out loud.

Dance or do sport

If you can get the chance to dance please do so. Dancing is great exercise and great fun. If you have ever fancied learning to ballroom dance, take this opportunity to get some lessons. Enjoy.

If you don't dance or don't want to dance,

Join a class or get a peer group

Whatever your age or current state of repair, there are classes and groups that walk together, dance together, cycle etc. Find some friends who like the same things or also want to control their weight and do things together. Go to an organised regular event or make up for your group (The Saturday morning riverside walk society).

Do what you used to enjoy doing

Remember when you did used to do a physical activity. It could be just walking or it could be tennis or Amateur Dramatics or painting or others. Find out about doing it again. Take your earlier passion and rediscover it.

In all of this, have an exercise plan and measure it. Decide what your exercise plan is going to be, write it down and measure how you do against it. Remember, lapses are OK. It is your plan and you can do whatever you like as long as you understand the consequences.

For those of you with an interest in getting a healthy heart or in getting fit, the following section will be of great interest to you.

I would ask anyone who is about to take any additional exercise and has any reason to believe that this may not be appropriate for them to talk to their medical practitioner before embarking on an exercise regime.

It is worth knowing what your various normal heart rates are. Carry out each of the following and note down your heart rate (take pulse at the end of each activity):

To take your heart rate, locate your pulse on your right wrist and count the number of beats over 30 seconds and then double that figure to get your heart rate in beats per minute.

- Standing - Stand quietly for 2 minutes.
- Sitting – Sit quietly for 2 minutes.
- Lying Down – Lie quietly for 2 minutes
- Taking a Walk – Take a five minute walk
- Talking to a friend – after talking for a few minutes
- Eating comfort food – Take pulse 5 minutes after you have finished eating
- Eating a meal – Just before you eat
- Eating a meal – 5 minutes after you have finished eating
- Ingesting caffeine – measure every minute for 10 minutes

Of course, you don't have to do the above in order to comply with our 12 day or 12 week rule. However, I think that you will find the results fascinating if you do it.

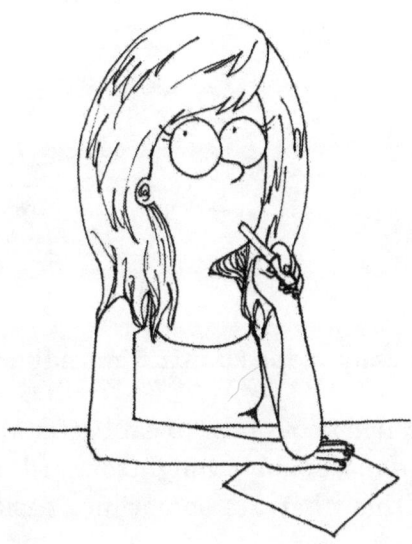

So how do we work out our maximum heart rate?

The reasonably accurate way is to take your age away from 220. So for me at 55, my maximum heart rate would be 165. For a 20 year old it would be 200.

If you want to be absolutely accurate with this, there is an excellent way of doing it accurately contained in Appendix 2.

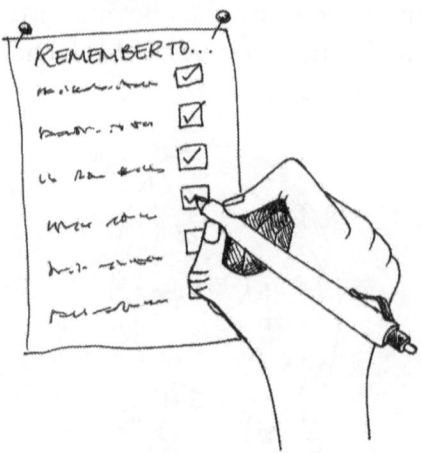

The 6 easy steps to mind management

So far I have explained about how to eat better and exercise better and both these are reasonably straightforward. However, as with many things like this, they are sometimes easier to say than to do.

But if you really want to achieve control over your weight it will help to have control over your mind.

I explained the Mind Model earlier in the programme. Here I go into a bit more detail about how to control the various elements of our mind.

When you think you are hungry – drink. If you are still hungry – eat. You know all this.

At all other times, do not rely on willpower to stop you eating when you are not hungry, use the gentle yet powerful TFT algorithms for anxiety, addiction and urge to eliminate the urge or desire to eat. You will be surprised how good this makes you feel.

Imagination is the key

A famous sage once said "you cannot achieve anything unless you can imagine it first". This is probably one of the most important statements in this book because if you cannot imagine yourself controlling your weight, you cannot achieve it.

We can all imagine as I explained earlier in the book. We all do it differently and we all have our own ways of describing it. What I want you to do is to sit quietly somewhere where you are comfortable and away from distractions.

Close your eyes and imagine the future. This can be a few weeks from now or a few months from now but no longer than 6 months. How ever far it is in the future imagine what will be happening. See yourself in the future, a fitter, healthier you who is managing your weight successfully. How does that feel? Enough said.

Now, with that imagination in your mind, move into the you that you see there. Just imagine what it will feel like to be that you. Feel how you will feel and feel how you will look. Take on the confidence that you will have and the sense of achievement and happiness. How do you look in those old clothes you love but nearly discarded? How does it feel to take moderate exercise without the exhaustion?

You know that now you have started to control your weight all that can and will be yours in just few short days, you will be moving quickly towards achieving it. You know that you can do it and you believe it and you believe in you.

Believe in yourself

If you don't, who will? Every time you are tempted to say "I can't", remember...

I WANT TO, I WANT TO - I CAN, I CAN, I CAN - I WILL and I HAVE

Understand where you are now and where you really want to be

You have done a lot of work to get to here. You know where you are. You know what you want to achieve and you know where your starting point is. You have been honest in this and you know exactly what you want to do.

There is no point kidding your conscious mind because it is the unconscious mind that will make the difference for you and it knows everything about you and you cannot lie to it.

Now you need to harness the fantastic strength you have in your unconscious mind for your benefit.

You have set down your objectives. Consistently and regularly review these and make sure that they stay appropriate to you what you want at that time.

Commit to yourself and to the journey step by step

Will Rogers once said "Even on the right track, you will still get run over if you just sit there"

From today you will commit to your plan and to the journey and you will commit to the vision you have of yourself in future, in the very near future.

Don't cheat on yourself

Remember that it is OK to lapse. If you cheat yourself, you are only cheating you.

Be truthful to yourself and accept the truth for what it is – real feedback is about you and what you really want.

One of the keys to any successful project is relaxed concentration. What you need here is to ensure you concentrate on getting the job done without any stress.

You already know how to feel good for absolutely no reason whatsoever.

You know the music you like and you know that relaxes you. Always have that music to hand so that you can trigger off your relaxation at any time. When you feel a 'stress – comfort food' trigger coming on or any time you feel your enthusiasm waning use the TFT algorithms and then listen to the music to make sure you relax fully.

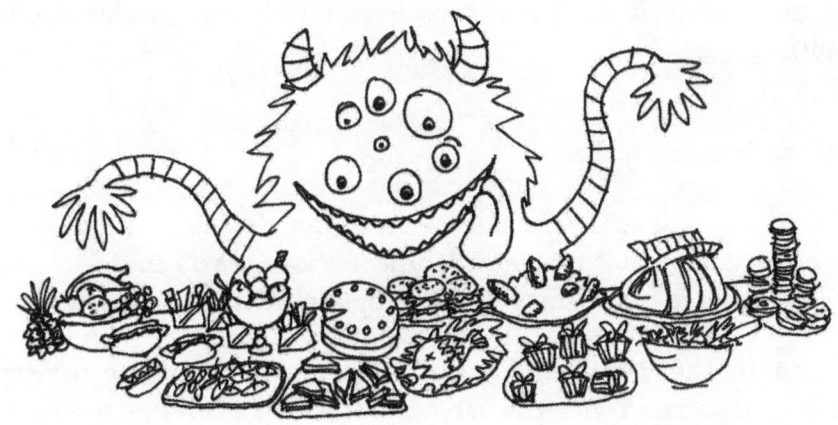

In the sections above, you have everything you need to control your weight successfully. However, there is still the question of habits. So this section adds even more powerful muscle to your system. Following this will mean having no excuses for not reaching your objectives.

Breaking Old Habits and Creating New Ones

Notice that I do not refer to habits as good or bad. Habits are formed for positive reasons and for our good. However, over time, the reasons can change and become inappropriate (going from childhood to adulthood) but we omit to change the habit to be appropriate.

In this section we will cover how to break old habits and create new ones.

Review of the Mind Model

We know that imagination is more powerful than willpower.

We know that our unconscious mind will not knowingly allow us to do anything that will harm us, so we have to educate it.

We know that it is the unconscious mind that produces our habits.

How to break a habit

It is quite simple really because when we don't do something every time there is a habit trigger, the unconscious starts to delete the habit and after a few times it will completely delete the habit.

We can use the craving and anxiety algorithms to ease the anxiety feelings associated with the habit and this will accelerate the habit breaking process.

It is hard to break a habit if the mind believes that there is a benefit in carrying on with it. Therefore, we need to substitute some benefit of equal or greater value in its place without needing the habit. That is, we need to fill the void physical or psychological left by deleting the habit. We also need to ensure we fill the void with something positive.

This is why feeling good for no reason is great. And also this is why visualising the future you and the benefits that will bring is so important to the success of this programme.

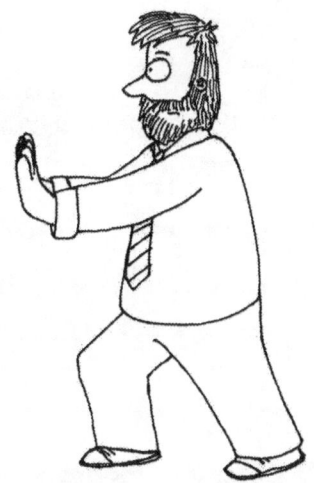

How to break a habit

Snacking

You know why you snack. You know why you eat when you are not hungry. So....stop it.

If you are hungry – have a drink of water. If you are still hungry – eat some proper food. Eat it only in the eating room.

If you are stressed, bored, anxious, upset, in need of comfort or whatever – tap the feeling away with the appropriate TFT algorithm and then feel good for no reason, think about that future you, have a drink, eat an apple. Use all your support groups, websites, buddies, family, anything to stop snacking.

Always start with correcting your PR (tap side of hand 15 times) then e, c, a, c, 9g, sq and if this does not work try c, e, c, 9g, sq. Other algorithms are in Appendix 3.

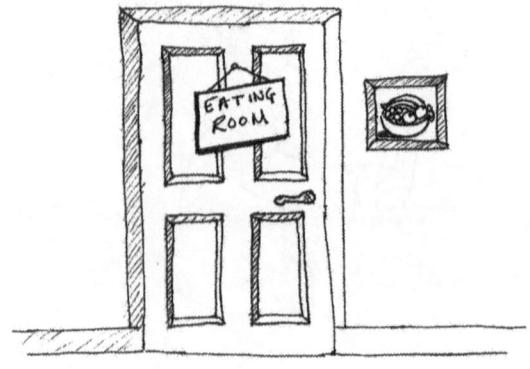

Eating anywhere

Only eat in the eating room.

Being lazy

Walk places. If a habit trigger comes – go for a brisk walk. If this doesn't have the required effect, use the algorithms. Do some housework, clean the car, mow the lawn. You know what to do.

Meal times

No set meal times. Even if the rest of the family eat at 7pm, you eat only when you are hungry and where do you eat? In the eating room only.

Waste bins

Remember that you do not have to finish everything on your plate. Decide the most appropriate waste bin.

The old habits of childhood are not appropriate now.

Being too hard on yourself

Be you own best friend, be encouraging, be supportive and most of all be really proud of yourself.

Creating a habit

If we repeat something over and over again, the unconscious processes it as a habit. The conscious mind does not then have to concern itself with it as the unconscious will instigate the habit based on the normal triggers.

A smoker, for example, who smokes 20 cigarettes a day for 20 years will have smoked 146,000 cigarettes. Enough I would say to form a particularly strong habit. In fact, the habit was probably formed by the time they had consumed their 100th cigarette. It doesn't take the mind long to recognise a pattern.

The smoker may have started at a young age in order to fit in with their friends, or to look older or another logical and reasonable reason. But, I bet, that their first cigarette was not a pleasurable experience. However, the other benefits were more important at the time than health or enjoyment.

Twenty years on are these reasons still appropriate? Probably not. We need to let our mind know this so we can break the habit. In fact it may be more like an addiction. For addictions we will need to treat ourselves with the TFT algorithms for addictive urge and anxiety. I covered these earlier and you can find them listed in Appendix 3. If you find these to be unsuitable for you, log onto www.oh-crikey.com and download additional help.

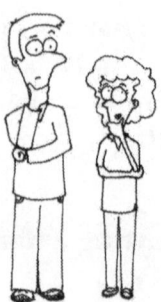

Things to do and think

Let's create some new habits that are appropriate to us now.

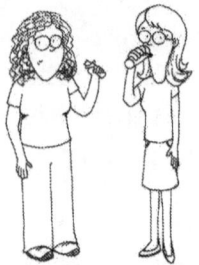

Snack on Water

Drink as much fresh water as you can without drowning in it.

Carry water with you and sip it often.

When you are hungry – eat

Please eat when you are sure that you are hungry. Please ignore set meal times.

Chew your food

Chew for the longest you can on each mouthful. This is obviously difficult with soup.

When you are satisfied – stop

When you are satisfied or start to feel full – please stop.

There is no food shortage. You do not need to finish everything. There will be more food later, when you are hungry again.

Shop only on a full stomach
Always eat in the Eating Room

Feel proud of yourself – you deserve it.

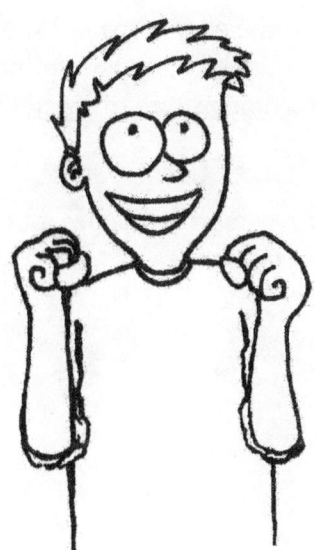

We have covered very many elements

- You know why you eat
- You know why you eat when you are not hungry
- You know about how anxiety affects your eating habits
- You know about weight management
- You know how you can control your weight and what doesn't work
- You have planned what you want to achieve and when
- You know how you will measure your success

- You are committed to achieving your objectives
- You have learned about Energy Meridian Systems
- You have learned about Thought Field Therapy ® and how you can use its powerful techniques to eliminate Anxiety.
- You have learned about Psychological Reversal and how to reverse it
- You now know about Individual Energy Toxins (IETs), how important they are to you (to eliminate them), how to identify and treat them
- You have learned how to self-administer TFT algorithm treatments
- You have covered the easy steps to weight management
- You have covered the easy steps to exercise management
- You have covered the easy steps to mind management
- You have covered many more tips and ideas that will help you succeed

To finalise your system we will discuss how to set up the best support structure that you can.

Chapter 10
Creating a great support structure

Family and friends

Tell everyone you have regular contact with what your objectives are and ask them to support you.

Explain to your partner/children how your system will work and ask them to support you in this for example, strange meal times (when you are hungry).

Colleagues

Ask colleagues at work to support and encourage you.

Online

Join our Yahoo Support Group and correspond by email with others using the system. You can join the group by requesting to via my website at www.oh-crikey.com

Training and instruction to help tap your cravings away is available via my website at www.oh-crikey.com.

You

Make sure you maintain your toxin diary

Make sure you keep practicing your TFT algorithms and treat yourself for PR regularly throughout the day.

Your imagination is stronger than your will, so keep imagining the new you and all the benefits you will receive from achieving your objectives.

Training

Join us on a 1-day course that goes through all the practical side of the book in detail. You can find out about these courses at www. oh-crikey.com

Contact us direct

You can contact us for support via my website at www.oh-crikey. com

At this point you need the system to start working for you, so I will condense all the above into a method that you can use to build your own successful weight management system.

Chapter 11
Your very own Weight Management System

To make it easy to see how the system will work we have summarised all the above into the following 4 sets of 6 easy steps. This should be used as your guideline for your weight management system. In addition to this, we ask you to use the TFT algorithms we have shown you to support your objectives.

The 6 easy steps to weight management

- When you think you are hungry – drink (key)
- When you are hungry – eat (key)
- Eat what your (detoxed) body tells you it needs
- Eat purposefully – enjoy every mouthful (key)
- When you are not hungry – stop eating (key)
- It's OK to lapse

The 6 easy steps to exercise management

- Walk places (a few minutes a day) (key)
- Use the stairs
- Dance or do sport
- Laugh more (key)
- Join a class/get a peer group
- Do what you used to enjoy doing

The 6 easy steps to mind management

- Use your TFT skills fully to help you succeed (key)
- Imagination is the key
- Believe in yourself (key)
- Know where you are and where you really want to be
- Commit to yourself (key)
- Don't cheat on you (key)

The 6 bits of other stuff that will help

- Ignore meal times where possible
- Shop only on a full stomach
- Shop only for today – if possible
- Put your cutlery down between bites (key)
- Have an eating room (key)
- Read food labels

There are over 30 system elements and we have summarised them in the 24 above. For the first 12 days and preferably for the first 12 weeks use the 12 key items noted above as your minimum system. If you can follow more of them - great. The more elements you follow, the greater the effect you will see and the sooner you will see it.

At all times use your support system to encourage and support you.

Basic TFT Algorithms

Use the TFT skills you now have to break bad habits and cravings. After this, use the parts of the system that suit your needs and objectives. If you follow the basic 12 from 24 activities labeled as key above, you will succeed in controlling your weight in line with your objectives.

Useful downloads

There are some useful forms and procedures you can get from me via my website at www.oh-crikey.com

A spreadsheet for measuring your success with your system elements is available. The spreadsheet enables you to track which elements you have successfully completed each day and gives you an easy to see view of your progress.

System design and conclusion

While you get used to the system and are experiencing the differing elements we have covered, we have put together a basic guideline system for you.

Once you are comfortable with the elements you can change this to suit your lifestyle and objectives.

Chapter 12
The next steps

Here is a basic system to follow to get you started.

1st 12 hours

Use this book and your success book

- Fill in your goals and targets and remind yourself everyday of your objectives and your progress by updating the booklet
- Identify your realistic and achievable goals
- Identify a reasonable time scale to achieve your objectives
- Make a milestone achievement plan (what to achieve each day or week or month that fits with your objectives)
- List the help and facilities that you will need to succeed
- Start developing your toxin diary
- Practise the treatment for PR
- Practise and use your TFT techniques
- List out your support structure
- Commit 100% to your plan
- Join the Yahoo Support Group

You can get access to the Yahoo site by requesting it via my website at www.oh-crikey.com

Use which waste bin?

When you know you are not hungry, decide where the waste bin is? In your mouth or under the sink or in the yard?

Imagine the future you

Everyday, whenever you have the chance to do it safely, bring back that vision of the future you. Feel how it good it feels to be that future you. Do I need to say more?

Fill your time and not your stomach

Get busy, do interesting stuff, do your own thing, get a buddy, go for a walk, dance, laugh, imagine the future you, play a CD. Do anything to not eat (as long as you are not hungry). Put together a list of the things you keep putting off and do them.

1st 12 days

- Take it one day at a time
- Review the 12 hour process – feel proud
- You know what's good for you
- Read sections of the book to re-enforce techniques
- Keep testing your foods for IETs and maintain your toxin diary
- Test for and treat PR regularly
- Practice and use your TFT algorithms
- Follow your plan
- Visit the Support Group
- Maintaining commitment
- What to do with a slip up. Do nothing, accept it and get on with putting it right by doing the right thing.
- Measure what you do
- Feel really proud of yourself

1st 12 weeks

- Maintain the 4 Key principles of eating
- Maintain the 2 Key principles of exercise
- Maintain the 4 Key principles of Mind Management

- Maintain the 2 other Key principles
- Keep testing for toxins
- Keep testing and treating for PR
- Average the rest on a two weekly basis. That is, try to keep to them but if not make sure you do every other week.
- Measure yourself on a weekly basis
- Fell proud and start to feel better every week
- And feel good, because you deserve to.

The rest of your life

Now, for the rest of your life you have a system that will work for you. Once you have used it for a few weeks you will create a good habit and soon you will not realise that you are doing many of the elements automatically.

If you have any concerns please contact me and I will be very pleased to help in any way I can.

It worked for me and I know that it will work for you. I look forward to hearing great success stories from you in the near future.

Success to you

Chapter 13
Personal Message from Steve

I have always been a sportsman but between the ages of 35 and 55, I let myself go. I played golf but did little else. My daughter was growing up, I was building my business. Business lunches, dinners, fast food, not enough time at home and a lack of exercise resulted in my weight management going out of the window.

I tried a number of diets and eating plans but got very disillusioned because they all seemed either something you could only do temporarily and would only have a temporary effect; or they were things you would need to do for life that revolved around deprivation and starvation.

So, I was stumped. I could, of course, do loads of exercise and lose the weight that way. But for how long could I do this? Until I was eighty?

The only plan that made any sense to me was to take the good bits from the common sense principles we are all brought up with like eat if you are hungry, chew your food properly, eat a balanced diet and keep active.

Then to add to that the useful bits and pieces from the good books I had read, like Paul McKenna's 'I Can Make You Thin' and other authors' similar works. Take a very large chunk out of Dr Roger Callahan's book 'Why do I eat when I am not hungry' and then find a way of cementing all this together with my own experiences into something that would work for me but fit my current lifestyle.

I needed no deprivation, no scolding and no starving. I needed a plan that let me eat when I was hungry and let me eat what my body told me to eat. I needed a plan that didn't require unusual levels of willpower. I also needed a plan that would let me lapse with no lasting effect physically or psychologically.

I found that the key element in achieving this was TFT and its techniques created and developed by Dr Callahan. Once I understood these, I knew that I had developed the most flexible, powerful and successful weight management system I knew of.

For every one of us who can get to control our weight, it is one healthier person and one good role model for the young.

I am now managing my weight perfectly. For all of you who follow the guidelines we have shown you in the book, I guarantee that you cannot fail to manage your weight successfully. The level of success will depend on how much commitment you have and the reasonability of your objectives.

I wish you all every success - thank you

Steve McNulty

Chapter 14
Contacts and web links

To get downloads related to this book and other good things on personal development

Oh Crikey Limited   www.oh-crikey.com

Callahan Techniques®   www.tftrx.com

To register for training in Weight Management

www.oh-crikey.com

To find training in TFT

Oh Crikey Limited   www.oh-crikey.com

Callahan Techniques®   www.tftrx.com

Association for Thought   www.atft.org

Field Therapy (ATFT)

To contact us

Use the email links on either of the websites above

Appendices

Appendix 1

Introduction to Callahan Techniques® Thought Field Therapy®

In the earlier parts of the book we have used TFT effectively to help us eliminate cravings and anxiety, to help us eliminate the need to mask these feelings by eating unnecessarily and to help us in controlling our weight.

TFT is an incredibly powerful therapy that can help you in every area of your life and I would strongly recommend you to study it further.

The creator of TFT, Dr Roger Callahan, has kindly produced this brief chapter explaining TFT in more detail. I know that this will interest you and I highly recommend his books, tapes and DVDs for further reading, especially the book 'Stop the Nightmares of Trauma' is invaluable if you want to take control of your life and also help those around you.

Roger's chapter is the 'TFT' part of the book. It explains some parts of Callahan Techniques® Thought Field Therapy® (TFT) which is where the key to this wonderfully successful weight management system came from and how, if you want to, you can use it to transform every area of your life and that of your nearest and dearest.

This chapter in the book contains some technical stuff and you will probably need to read it a couple of times for some of the ideas to sink in. Don't worry about this – it is a natural process and will be well worth it. We have made references to other books and training courses that you can refer to if you want more detailed information.

This section can be a serious positive influence on the rest of your life. So let's hand over to Dr Roger Callahan.

Callahan Techniques® Thought Field Therapy® (TFT)
Dr Roger Callahan PhD

Energy Meridians

The ancient eastern civilisations discovered the acupuncture meridians over 3,000 years ago and treatments such as Acupuncture and Chakra based therapies have developed using them.

Many in the scientific world now accept totally the existence of energy meridians in the body. Some scientists have used sophisticated scanning equipment to capture them in pictures.

The meridians flow around our body using the major organs and vessels as conduits and 'stopping off' points. They are symmetrical on the body and are an important element in the body's well-being.

With all energy systems, they rely on electrical current. Every piece of matter in the universe has a form of electrical energy associated with it. Even a lump of stone is held together by electricity at the atomic level.

All electrical systems have positive and negative elements and, depending on the strength of each, the system will either flow positively or negatively.

It will come as no surprise to you that when you are unhappy, your energy drops and when you are really happy you have loads of energy. So we know that how we feel affects our physical systems.

It is a known fact that when we have a negative disposition, our energy is low and our energy meridian is flowing negatively.

It is also known that if we can change the flow to positive it helps us feel better.

When we are ill or emotionally upset our energy systems do not flow properly, are negatively charged and we can fail to think clearly.

I developed TFT by finding certain defined spots in the acupuncture system. This is the basis for curing the problems.

This section will show you how to use this accurate tapping technique to reduce your anxiety based eating, stop your food addictions and cravings, eliminate the need to eat when you are not hungry and, if used with the system we propose, will give you total control over your weight and your life for evermore.

Remember, when we ask you to tap, **tap at least 10 times** (more if we define the number) on the spot requested. Tap hard enough to put some energy into the system but not nearly hard enough to hurt yourself.

A brief history of TFT

A theory to be on-line with reality must *begin* with reality. TFT theory is *inductive*. Induction is the process of making generalizations from observations. These generalisations are the essence of scientific discovery. Without them, people could not learn from experience *(Peikoff, 2002)*.

In the context of TFT, this means that I began my discoveries with sensory-based observations of actual phenomena (I watched what happened when I did things with my tapping sequences). The principles discussed in this section came directly from those observations.

I developed TFT theory by conducting repeatable first-hand experiments. Initially, I observed that when my client, Mary, tapped under her eye, her lifelong and previously unresponsive severe phobia of water was completely cured.

Although I had been studying Applied Kinesiology and the concept of energy meridians, I made this observation without any pre-existing thoughts about the therapy that I applied, which I had yet to name Thought Field Therapy®.

After my success with Mary, I repeated this with a number of my clients; however, I observed that most of them did not respond to this one point treatment for phobias. This did not negate what I initially observed with Mary, who clearly had her phobia cured as a result of tapping under her eye. What I did at this time was to find combinations of other points that would help such people. I also used my previous discovery of a correction for what I called Psychological Reversal (PR). When I applied this PR correction, my success rate nearly doubled. PR treatment is the process by which we can literally change the direction of the energy flow in our body from Negative to Positive. We cover this later in detail later.

I continued to make further discoveries in order to refine and increase the power of TFT further.

You will be learning about some of these discoveries in this section. I discovered much more by using my development of Voice Technology, with approximately a 97-98% success rate. These results are comparable to those achieved in the hard sciences of Chemistry and Physics. The method we will show you in this section will give you a 70%-90% success rate in reducing your eating when you are not hungry. It will also show you how to treat yourself for other anxiety based life issues.

How TFT Differs from Other Approaches

The truth or accuracy of a theory can best be determined by the results it produces. In simple terms "the proof of the pudding is in the eating" - quite apt for our subject. The real test for the validity of a theory is whether or not that theory is on-line with reality. In developing TFT, I began with direct observation, developed theoretical principles and concepts, and continued to experiment and observe the results.

TFT produces, in a very high percentage of cases, total elimination of all traces of psychological distress (emotional upset). This works for issues such as trauma, stress, depression, anxiety, pain, rage, anger etc.

TFT does not do anything directly to the brain nor to its biochemistry. It does nothing to change core beliefs, and people are not required to relive their childhood experiences. It does not make people suffer more pain than they want to or thought they could.

What TFT does is provide a code for eliminating emotional upset at its root cause. Emotional upset can be mild as in a few minutes boredom or can be very harsh as in a life-long trauma.

A therapy that is truly deep and addresses the root causes of psychological distress ought to be able to produce real change in people and thereby eliminate the problem.

TFT does just that.

In doing so, it revolutionizes the field. The best way for you to see this is to begin using TFT with any anxiety you feel and observe the profound changes that occur as you eliminate it. We will show you how to do this.

As you do, you will see that the results of successful Thought Field Therapy® are indeed occurring at the deepest, most fundamental level possible.

A formal definition of Callahan Techniques® Thought Field Therapy® (TFT) could be:

TFT is a treatment which provides a code, that when applied to a problem to which the individual is attuned (thinking about), will eliminate upsets in the thought field. Upsets in the thought field are the fundamental cause of all negative emotions.

We will be using a lot of terms, definitions and instructions when teaching you on how to use TFT. We ask you to take what we say and apply it immediately without questioning it or its basis for working. You will be amazed.

However, we do not expect you to then continue to blindly follow our every suggestion. We only want you to firstly convince yourself that it works – not how it works.

Nothing we ask you to do can harm you. Nothing is intrusive, is drug based, and is any form of hypnotism or other diversion. The worst you can leave with is being the same as when you started.

We expect you to feel better as you experience TFT more and more as we progress through the book.

Explanations for some of the things that we ask you to do can be found in the appendices to this book. For a deeper understanding of TFT, how it works and how you can use it for all areas of your life and that of your loved ones; I suggest reading my book 'Stopping the nightmares of trauma'.

Thought Fields

In TFT, the word, "thought field," can often be used interchangeably with the words, "memory," or simply "thought;" however, in order to understand the dynamics of TFT, it is helpful to think of a memory in terms of a thought field, for these fields contain the causes of the upsets that cause our emotional distress. We call these causes 'perturbations'. So when we talk about a perturbation in the thought field we are talking about an exquisitely detailed body of information that causes the physiological results that we are aware of in a disturbing emotion.

We know that it is the perturbation in the thought field that causes the upset because this is the part of the problem which is collapsed with successful treatment.

If someone were to enter the room and tell you that you had just won 10 million dollars in the lottery, you would be in a different thought field from the one you are in now. Your body would begin secreting chemicals that would change the way you feel.

A field is an invisible, non-material structure in space that has an effect upon matter. You cannot go out and buy 1 lb of thought or a bunch of thought. It has no substance.

Michael Faraday, a self-schooled genius of science, introduced the concept of a field. Faraday called attention to the fact that although one cannot see, feel, or taste an electromagnetic field, one will be able to see its effects if iron filings are placed on a piece of paper with a magnet under it. The iron filings clearly show the outline, in two dimensions, of the three-dimensional field.

Another invisible field is the gravitational field. While we can't see it, we can see its effects when we drop a rock and watch it fall to the ground. In fact, fields are all around us. Every living being generates electromagnetic fields that can be measured as far as several feet away from the body. Moreover, cell phones depend on fields in order to work, and gravitational fields keep the planets orbiting around the sun.

When a person only becomes upset when he or she tunes into a memory, which is a thought field that contains perturbations, these perturbations become activated through the body's energy system. The person will then feel psychological effects and perhaps even physiological effects that were caused by the perturbations in the thought field. As the person taps using the TFT system and coding, putting carefully selected energy into the system, the perturbations in the thought field are collapsed, changing the chemical make-up of the body. As a result, the person feels better.

Although thought fields and perturbations are not energy in and of themselves, they require energy for activation. The body's energy system is activated and comes into play when the person tunes into the emotional problem or upset. For every energy meridian point on the body that is being treated, a perturbation is being eliminated. As a result, the person is freed from psychological distress.

Further information on Thought Fields can be found my book 'Tapping the Healer within'.

Perturbations

In essence, when you treat yourself with TFT, you are collapsing perturbations that are encoded in the particular thought field associated with the problem on which you are focusing. A perturbation (P) is defined as "a subtle, but clearly isolable aspect of a thought field that is responsible for triggering and controlling all negative emotions."

P's are Isolable

It is important to note that the perturbation is *isolable*. Isolable means that the treatment removes only the problem causing information and not other important information in the thought field. This means when the perturbation collapses, along with the information causing the problem, the problem will be removed. The memory of the experience and what the person learned as a result will remain. Not like people who take the drug LSD, for example, which can cure the fear of heights, as it is dangerous because a good many people jump out of windows when they take LSD.

Contrary to popular and professional belief, it is not the memory of a trauma that causes problems for a person. The problem is the activation of the perturbation, which sets off a chain of biochemical and psychological events for the person whenever he/she voluntarily or involuntarily focuses on the problem.

After a successful TFT treatment, the person can think about a previously upsetting traumatic event without any trace of emotional upset. In some cases, the memory can even become more clear and detailed than it was prior to treatment, but without the distress.

Active Information

Perturbations contain "active INFORMATION" that is activated and amplified when the thought field is attuned when the person thinks about the problem. The emotional problem can then be treated through stimulation of the proper energy meridian points.

Causal Diagnosis— *How TFT Algorithms Were Discovered*

The next obvious question would be, *"How do we know which energy meridian points on the body to address and in what sequence?"* In other words, how were the algorithms discovered?

An Algorithm is a sequence of points in a defined order to treat a specific issue. They are a bit like a road map or set of directions. That is, they must be followed carefully and exactly to have the full effect required.

The specific points used to treat various problems were discovered through my causal diagnostic procedures. When a person is being treated with a TFT algorithm, specific energy meridian points are stimulated (using a tapping technique) in an exact, predetermined sequence.

Through the stimulation of the correct treatment points in the correct sequence, the perturbation is collapsed. As a result, all traces of psychological distress (emotional upset) are eliminated at their root cause.

Much like a combination lock, *the correct sequence is crucial to the success of the treatment.* If you had a correct combination (code) on a lock of 3-27-32-5, and you tried to open the lock with a changed sequence (27-32-5-3, for instance), the lock wouldn't open. The same is true with the codes for TFT algorithms. Keep in mind that if an important treatment does not work for you, you need to find a person trained in causal diagnosis who can discover exactly what you need.

The TFT algorithms were developed, *not* by random trial and error, but through the use of a causal diagnostic procedure that reveals which meridian points to stimulate and in what order. I found that order can be very important and since there are 14 possible TFT treatment points, providing over 87 billion possible treatment combinations; this means that these algorithms could not have been developed by chance. Mathematically, if you started trying out possible treatment point combinations in the year of Christ's birth and continued without taking any breaks at all, you would still have approximately 163,800 more years to go!

I found that a particular sequence worked for high percentages (80-90%) of people, after I had treated hundreds of people with a particular psychological problem, this sequence became an algorithm. Someone who has been trained in TFT diagnosis or especially Voice Technology can usually successfully treat the 10-20% of people for whom the algorithms do not work.

The outcome of TFT algorithm treatment can easily be replicated by anyone who learns the algorithms and applies them correctly, with the same high success rate.

By reading this book, you will learn to replicate these rapid, painless, and highly successful treatments. By practicing the techniques, you will learn the skills necessary to treat negative emotions and conditions previously thought to be incurable.

When you use these treatments and see their results, you will learn that TFT theory can be tested in reality and put to immediate practical use. Hence, we can say with assurance that TFT theory is *on-line with reality*!

How Change is Measured in TFT

The Subjective Units of Distress Scale (SUD)

SUD is an abbreviation for the useful term, "Subjective Units of Distress." This scale provides a way to quantify the degree of stress, pain, or disturbing emotions experienced.

The SUD may be represented on an 11-point or 10-point scale, 0 to 10 or 1 to 10, respectively. That is, when you are upset you would rate it on a scale of 1 to 10 with 1 being not upset to 10 being totally as upset as you could possibly be.

In TFT, the SUD is considered the "bottom line" by which therapy is evaluated for success. Behavioural indices of how people are responding to therapy may be quite misleading, since many people can do most things when pushed. If their suffering remains intense at the same time, we do not consider this to be successful therapy.

As in the case of Mary, she had learned from conventional therapy that she could withstand a great deal more suffering than she thought she originally could. Once she had been successfully treated with TFT, all traces of her water phobia had disappeared, including her weekly nightmares of water 'getting her'.

You can also observe physiological changes after successful TFT treatment, such as changes in:

- skin colour – *healthy colour comes into face*

- breathing rate - *becomes less rapid and more deep*
- facial expression - *becomes visibly more relaxed*
- body language - *posture changes from "closed" to "open," and the body becomes more relaxed*
- body temperature - *may rise or fall slightly*
- pulse rate - *often significant reduction if it is high*
- blood pressure - *often significant reduction if it is high*

The most important physiological changes are unprecedented improvements in Heart Rate Variability (HRV).

The Apex Problem

The apex problem is the tendency for people to fail to recognize that the TFT treatment was responsible for eliminating their problem. At times, even though people recognize that their troubling symptoms are no longer present, they do not attribute this change to TFT. In some cases, people can even forget that they ever had the problem! TFT can bring results so immediate that it is often beyond their comprehension that TFT could actually have cured their problem. Some typical statements that indicate an apex problem are:

- "I can't think of it right now." (People often say this when they are asked for a post-treatment SUD.)
- "You distracted me." (This one is *very* common!)
- "I know it will come back as soon as I leave here."
- "I can't remember what I was thinking about."
- "This is too simple. It couldn't have worked."
- "I really wasn't that afraid."
- "I have worked on this for years. This couldn't have made the difference."
- "This treatment repressed my feelings."
- "It's really not the kind of thing you can give a SUD rating to." (People can say this even though they had no trouble giving a high SUD rating before treatment.)

The Apex Problem can sabotage further treatment. It is, therefore, important to be aware of it.

If you do not recognize the effectiveness of TFT due to the apex problem, you might not continue using TFT and this can serious affect the effectiveness of your weight management system.

Cure and Time

People often ask us about the cures associated with TFT, "How long will it last?" We normally respond "As long as you follow what we ask you to do". However, there are some things that you need to be aware of.

Once a perturbation in a thought field is collapsed, will it remain? I have discovered what can bring back a successfully treated problem – it is what I call an Individual Energy Toxin (IET).

IETs are distinguished from the more general toxins such as lead, mercury, cadmium, arsenic by the fact that they represent an **individual's** sensitivity to certain common foods such as wheat, milk, eggs, etc. It can be demonstrated that such foods affect the energy (testing) system first. IETs can be treated (usually **not** cured) by treating the individual and this evidently lowers the threshold of the toxin for a while. If you wish to find out more about your IETs contact your local Diagnostic or VT practitioner who can be found in the membership directories at www.tftrx.com and www.atft.org

What can bring a problem back?

- Energy Toxins (covered in the next chapter)
- A new, similar trauma

Is there a time limit? No, it depends on you but we will guide you.

Can it be re-eliminated? Yes, we will show you how and you will have all the tools to deal with it.

The exception to this is the addiction algorithm, which commonly needs to be repeated every time the client gets the urge for what he/she is addicted to.

Individual Energy Toxins (IETs)

What is an Individual Energy Toxin?

The identification of IETs and their elimination will take you well over half way to achieving your weight management objectives. Therefore, it is extremely important that you read this section over and over until you understand it. More explanation is given on our website at www.tftrx.com

When TFT works and the emotional upset or the other problems are eliminated, then a cure has occurred. In most cases, this cure will be lasting. In some cases, the cure will be undone, and the perturbations and symptoms will manifest again.

After working with many of these situations, I discovered that the cause of this undoing was an exposure to a substance to which the person reacted negatively, at the energy level.

These substances may be found in everyday life situations and are harmless to most individuals. For some individuals, however, these substances can cause serious problems. Because these reactions are unique to individuals and affect these energy systems in specific ways, they are called Individual Energy Toxins (IETs).

Practitioners trained in TFT Diagnosis or TFT Voice Technology can identify IETs for you.

For the weight loss programme, we will teach you some basic methods of identification and treatment. For more advanced work and to see a really fantastic effect on your energy levels and positive outlook on life, You can also buy a kit from us, developed by me, called "Sensitivities, Intolerances, and TOXINS: How to Identify and Neutralize Them with TFT."

Some IETs might be expected, e.g., tobacco, pesticides, and various organic chemicals (in clothing, carpets, upholstery, paint, etc.); however, some of the most common IETs are unexpected, e.g., wheat, corn, eggs, milk and other dairy products, perfumes, laundry soap or detergents, scented tissue, shampoo, or deodorants.

The Barrel Effect

The barrel effect is an important factor in understanding toxins. Dr. Doris Rapp explained this very concisely in her video, *Environmentally Sick Schools*. The body deals with each suspect food, or other toxin, as if it were being contained in a barrel where it can be isolated before being disposed of. One toxin may not necessarily become a problem; however, if the barrel is filled to overflowing, then a problem can develop. The toxin spills over to exert a physiological or psychological effect on the body.

The size of the barrel will differ for each item and will also vary in size, according to each individual and his/her state of health. A very ill, weak person may be said to have a very small barrel in which to isolate toxins. A young, vigorous, and healthy person is likely to have larger barrel and can therefore tolerate greater exposure. When we know of an item that is toxic to us, e.g., wheat, our barrel size for that toxin will increase if we stay away from the toxin for two or three months. This explains why a person may indulge in a toxin for a short while with no apparent ill effects before those effects appear.

An interesting question is this—when someone treats a toxin, is he/she increasing the barrel size or actually removing the item from a list of potentially harmful items? The direct evidence of our standard approach in TFT suggests that we can indeed strengthen an individual (i.e., increase the size of the toxin barrel) with our treatments. We can eliminate problems, even though the person's problem might originate in toxin exposure.

This has been commonplace for many years. Dr. Arthur Coca (1994), in *The Pulse Test*, maintained that we do not become allergic by over-indulging in a particular substance. Instead, our allergens are determined by our heredity. In other words, he suggested that the barrel for some foods will never overflow unless that food was an inherited sensitivity.

Indicators of Toxic Sensitivity

- Malaise
- Water Retention
- Fidgeting/Restless Feet/Legs
- Hyperactivity/Labile Emotions
- Constipation/Diarrhoea
- Red Ears/Blotchy Skin (neurodermatitis)
- Sticky Faeces
- Fatigue after meals
- Panic Attacks
- Hyperactivity
- Insomnia
- Irritability
- Obesity
- Bloatedness
- Nausea
- Cravings (e.g. for specific foods)

So, from the above you can see the effect on the body that IETs have. They also stop the body operating effectively and add seriously to weight issues.

Can IETs be "cleared"?

We are often asked if the IETs themselves can be treated with TFT (or some other method) so that the person can continue to consume the identified substance without ill effects. Given that toxins can often be favourite foods, we all wish that this were so!

I and other Callahan Techniques® approved advanced TFT practitioners have experimented extensively with several so-called "toxin clearing" treatments and are aware of the extensive claims that are being made for a number of such methods. It has been our experience that these methods **do not** neutralize IETs to the point where a person can continue to consume a substance without the ill effects.

This can be extremely dangerous because some ill effects have *no apparent symptoms*, and the person incorrectly believes that the toxin has been "cleared." In fact, the toxin has not been cleared, and the person risks his/her health without even knowing it. This may only reveal itself when the person has become very ill, often too late for resolution to take place.

Since IETs can often be people's favourite foods (i.e., they have become addicted to the IET), they desperately want to believe that the toxicity can be "cleared" so they can continue to indulge. Hence, they can become susceptible to the false claims of those who say that they can clear toxins.

Once your problem has been eliminated you should continue to avoid toxins for at least two months while you are totally symptom free. After that you can re-introduce them with care. Contact your therapist or trainer at once if the symptoms return.

The Pulse Test

Arthur F. Coca, MD was a top allergist who founded the medical organization of allergists and edited the major journal. He was a Professor at Columbia University and was highly regarded in his profession until his discovery of the role of the pulse in identifying allergens. This simple test caused him to be ostracized.

Mrs. Coca was a medical researcher. She was hospitalized with angina and given only five years to live. Mrs. Coca was given a morphine derivative while in hospital, and her pulse began beating so fast that it could not be counted easily–faster than 180 beats per minute. Mrs. Coca mentioned that her pulse often raced after certain meals. This led to Dr. Coca to explore and find that the pulse increases with the ingestion of an allergen/toxin. He suggested that she count her pulse following the intake of SINGLE FOODS to see if other culprits might be identified.

He was able to experiment with many of his patients and to develop a simple and efficient means of identifying the substances, which affected the health of his patients. His small and readable book, *The Pulse Test*, is highly recommended for a full explanation of his theories and techniques. His Pulse Test is described in Appendix 2 of this book.

Proximity Toxins

A proximity toxin is any toxin in the immediate environment, such as the person's clothing, hair spray, perfume, smoke, or any other airborne substance, that enters the body via the lungs. I found that such toxins could completely prevent a treatment from working or holding, even in the short term. For an inhalant toxin, in the past, the clients would have to remove their clothing and put on a gown washed in a substance that was not toxic to them. They could also wear a surgical mask to prevent them from inhaling the toxic fumes. Another option was to have them shower and wash their hair before treating them with TFT. Fortunately, the correction described below will work about 80% of the time, making removal of the offending clothing, showering, or other radical change unnecessary.

I have recently determined that this correction will often work for an ingested toxin, as well.

Toxin Correction for difficult to treat PR

Tap the Index Finger 15 times.
Tap the Specific PR spot (side of hand) 15 times.
Then, repeat the treatment that hadn't previously worked.

The Components of some selected TFT Algorithms and the tapping sequences

Algorithms follow a standard well-defined pattern. By completing each step strictly in the order that they are prescribed, you will be performing effective TFT in a very efficient manner. There is one standard protocol for all Algorithms, and it conforms to the architecture commonly present in TFT. The places we will ask you to tap are shown in the following diagram

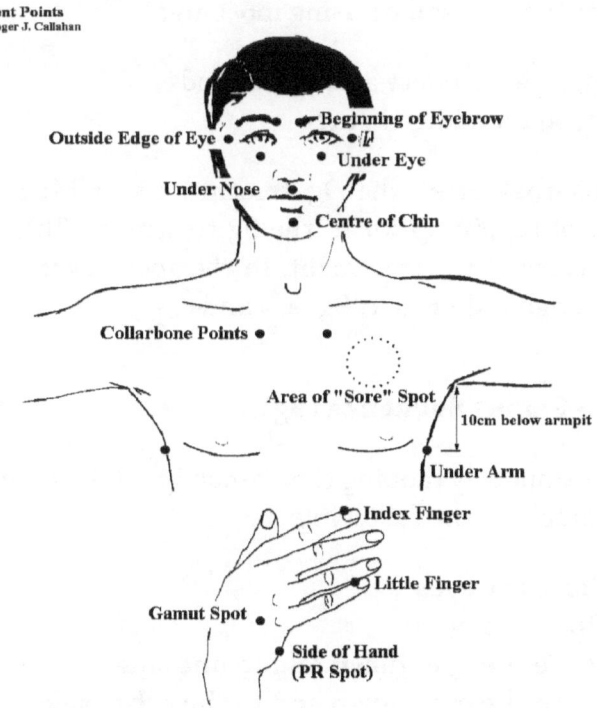

THE CALLAHAN
TECHNIQUES®

Treatment Points
© 1994 Roger J. Callahan

Beginning of Eyebrow

Outside Edge of Eye

Under Eye

Under Nose

Centre of Chin

Collarbone Points

Area of "Sore" Spot

10cm below armpit

Under Arm

Index Finger

Little Finger

Gamut Spot

Side of Hand
(PR Spot)

To illustrate this, the TFT protocol for the treatment of anxiety is shown below:

In an abbreviated form, it can be written: **e, a, c, 9g, sq.**

In TFT terminology this means under the eye, under the arm, collarbone, 9 gamut treatment and then repeating the first three again. We will cover all the abbreviations later.

The complete treatment sequence is known as a **Holon**.

TFT Algorithms for cravings

An algorithm is a recipe of one or more points which together comprise a treatment that has been found to work for a particular problem (such as anxiety or stress) in approximately 70% to 90% percent of cases. The simple algorithms and a guide to the abbreviations are listed in Appendix 3.

The algorithms we will be using most are:

E, a, c, 9g, sq for anxiety and stress, and
C, e, c, 9g, sq for addictive urge

Sq means that after the 9g treatment you MUST repeat the sequence of tapping prior to the 9g treatment. This is important to the success of the treatment. In the above example this would mean in longhand - E, a, c, 9g, e, a and c.

The Nine Gamut Sequence (9g)

While continuously tapping the Gamut Spot (allowing about 5 taps for each step), do the following:

1. **Close the eyes**
2. **Open the eyes**
3. **Move the eyes down and to one side**
4. **Move the eyes down and to the other side**

5. **Roll the eyes in a circle in one direction**
6. **Roll the eyes in a circle in the opposite direction**
7. **Hum a tune (about five notes) out loud**
8. **Count out loud from one to five**
9. **Hum a tune again aloud**

Steps 1 to 6 of the Nine Gamut Sequence can be performed in any order (i.e., eyes down left first or eyes down right first; eyes in a circle to the left first or eyes in a circle to the right first).

The Floor to Ceiling Eye Roll (Rapid Relaxation)

The floor to ceiling eye roll should be used at the end of all of the Algorithm treatments when the SUD is a 3 or lower. It will usually bring a SUD of 3 to a 1 (on a 10-point scale) or 0 (on an 11-point scale). If not, go back to where you were in the Protocol and do the next step.

Hold the head level, move the eyes (not the head) down to the floor. Tap the Gamut sport while you slowly raise the eyes to the ceiling.

This treatment can also be done by itself for the purposes of stress reduction or rapid relaxation.

Using the SUD (Subjective Units of Distress) Scale

The importance of individuals' report of their subjective level of pain (1 to 10 or 0 to 10) has been recognized as accurate and important in monitoring the health and recovery of hospitalized individuals. It is now required as a vital sign to monitor, along with heart rate, blood pressure, temperature, and breathing rate. Similarly, the most important measure of the power of TFT is *your report of your experience.*

The way we measure this is through the use of the Subjective Units of Distress (SUD) Scale. You are asked to rate their level of discomfort on a 10-point (1-10) scale or on an 11-point (0-10) scale.

Most individuals will quickly learn to use this tool to communicate the level of distress they are experiencing as they tune into a thought field.

While the 1 to 10-point scale is the most common self-report, *any* scale or description of graduated intensity is acceptable, as long as clients are able to be consistent in their report.

Be very clear with that 0 or 1 will represent no distress and 10 will represent maximum distress.

It is also important to emphasize you should come up with the number that best represents the degree of upset at this moment just thinking about the problem, **not** how you have felt in the past or how you anticipate you might feel in the future.

You will evaluate the SUD at specific points in the treatment, as outlined in the Protocol. You can compare the sensations in your body when you determine the SUD *during* the treatment with the sensations in your body when you *originally* gave evaluated the SUD. By doing so, you will be able determine if the SUD has changed.

Psychological Reversals and their Correction - The TFT Law of Reversal

Psychological Reversal (PR) is literally a state of reversed polarity in the body.

This state or condition blocks natural healing and prevents otherwise effective treatments from working. I discovered that a person who is in a state of psychological reversal is unable to respond to an otherwise effective TFT treatment or any other effective treatment.

A person can be psychologically reversed in just one, a select few, or many areas of life. For instance, a person who has a "mental block" against learning mathematics might be psychologically reversed only in that area and not with other subjects.

A person who is psychologically reversed in most or all domains in life is considered to be massively reversed. The PR state is usually accompanied by negative attitudes and self-sabotaging behaviour. Correction of psychological reversal is a vital step in successful treatment for people who are reversed.

An interesting symptom of PR is that concepts are reversed 180 degrees (e.g., people will say left when they mean right, South when they mean North, but not East when they mean North). They may also reverse numbers and/or letters. The common typing error of reversing letters can indicate that the typist is in a temporary state of PR.

In the 1940s, Langman (1972) discovered that 95% of the women in his study who had tumours that were not malignant showed a positive polarity when measured with a voltmeter, and 96% of the women who had tumours that were malignant showed a negative polarity (Burr, 1972).

All of the women had tumours, yet the polarity distinguished the cancer from the non-cancer. Complete removal of the tumour corrected the reversal of polarity. This was the only way they knew to correct a reversal. I have found a number of ways to correct a reversal. Blaich (1988) found that readers improved in reading speed by 45% after treating for reversal using my discoveries. Teachers have helped students who were writing backwards or reversing letters to write correctly.

How to Recognize a Psychological Reversal (PR)

- TFT or other treatments (e.g. a medical treatment that is normally effective) do not work
- Reversing words, concepts, and / or numbers
- Dyslexia (likely to be a massive reversal state)
- Grumpy, irritable, negative mood

- Self-sabotaging behaviour
- Negative self-talk
- Procrastination
- Having a "mental block" in a particular area, such as mathematics, writing, computers, etc
- Client does not respond to appropriate algorithm treatment and then responds to the same treatment after PR correction.

Once PR has been corrected, which is an extraordinarily simple process, approximately 80% of people who did not respond to a TFT treatment will report the expected decrease in SUD after they repeat the same treatment.

Psychological Reversal Corrections

At any level, once PR has been corrected, begin the algorithm again from the beginning.

Correction for Specific PR

Indication: *Little or no change in SUD after the majors*

Tap the Specific PR spot on the side of the hand (karate chop point) about 15 times while focusing on the problem.

Repeat the majors. Check SUD. If SUD has not dropped 2 or more points, go to Recurring PR (Appendix 1).

There are a number of other treatments for PR but for normal purposes, tapping the side of the hand (Karate Chop point) is usually sufficient.

Collarbone Breathing Treatment (CB2)

Collarbone breathing (CB2) is a treatment I developed that will often help a very resistant problem to respond to TFT treatments.

When doing Collarbone Breathing in the context of a TFT treatment for a particular problem, you must be tuned into the thought field of the issue being addressed.

I recommend that people working on addictions do CB2 at least three times a day, in addition to correcting their PR 15-20 times a day (side of hand, sore spot, and under nose).

Anxiety and Panic Disorders and Obsessive/Compulsive Disorders (OCD) need to do Collarbone Breathing three times a day and correct their PR 15-20 times a day (side of hand, sore spot, and under nose) on a regular basis.

In the Collarbone Breathing treatment below, when the knuckles touch the body, only they should touch the body.

Indications that Collarbone Breathing may be needed:

- TFT and / or PR Corrections won't work or won't hold.
- SUD is going down very slowly, i.e. 8, 7, 6, 5, 4, etc.
- Co-ordination is off, and the person is awkward.
- Person has unbalanced gait—arms don't swing evenly and smoothly when person walks (4% of people walk with one arm curtailed, and 2% of people walk with both arms curtailed).
- Person chronically reverses actions, concepts, and thoughts.
- Person is declining in performance and / or competence.
- Timing is off, and person is confused.
- Reading makes person yawn / feel sleepy
- Person is hyperactive.

THE COLLARBONE BREATHING EXERCISE
1993 Roger J. Callahan, PhD

What I call the "collarbone points" are located in the following way:

Go to the base of the throat, about where a man might knot his tie. From that point, feel for the notch in the centre of the collarbone. Go straight down about one inch, and the collarbone points are about one inch to the right and left of centre (see treatment point diagram).

BREATHING POSITIONS [START WITH NORMAL BREATHING]

There are five breathing positions in this exercise:

1. Take a deep breath in fully and hold it.
2. Let half of that breath out and hold it.
3. Let it all out and hold it.
4. Take a half breath in and hold it.
5. Breathe normally.

THE TOUCHING POSITIONS

1. Take two fingertips and touch one of the collarbone points and tap the gamut spot on the back of that hand while going through the 5 breathing positions. Tap rapidly with about 5 good taps for each of the five breathing positions.

2. Move the same two fingertips to the other collarbone point and repeat above.

3. Now, bend the same two fingers in half and touch the knuckles to the collarbone point while tapping and going through the five breathing positions. Either tuck the thumb in or keep it in the air. Make sure that the elbows are in the air when you are touching the

knuckles to the body so that only the knuckles are touching the body. The back of the hand is a negative polarity, so the treatment would not work if the thumb or elbow (positive polarities) were to touch the body.

4. Move knuckles to the other collarbone point and tap while going through the five breathing positions. Make sure that only the knuckles are touching the body.

5. Now, take fingertips of OTHER hand and repeat steps 1 and 2 above.

6. Now, take knuckles of that hand and repeat steps 3 and 4 above, making sure that only the knuckles are touching the body.

You have just done the 40 breathing and tapping exercises—20 with the fingertips, and 20 with the knuckles. You have done five breathing positions on eight touching positions. Please learn to do these well so that you are able to do them automatically.

The TFT tapping technique - using TFT Algorithms

When we get an addictive urge with food or we get anxiety based cravings or desires for food and we know that we are not hungry, we can tap away these desires/cravings/urges using the tapping techniques of TFT.

This gives us tremendous power in managing our weight. When we collapse and eliminate the anxiety, we have no need to mask anything and therefore we do not need to change our feelings and so we have no need to eat (unless we are really hungry).

You are now in more control.

Key to Abbreviations for TFT Algorithm Treatment Points

SUD subjective **u**nits of **d**istress (a rating on a scale of 0-10 or 1-10 of how upset one is at the moment)

e under **e**ye (under the pupil just below the rim of the bone—the inside of the tip of the second toe on the side of the large toe also works if the person is not able to tap on the face)

a under **a**rm (about 4 inches down from the arm pit; in the middle of the bra line for women)

c collarbone (1 inch down from the V of the neck, and 1 inch over to either the left or right side)

eb eye**b**row (at the point where the eyebrow begins, near the nose—the outside of the small toe also works if the person is not able to tap on the face)

if index **f**inger (beside the nail on the side toward the thumb)

oe outside of **e**ye (about ½ inch straight out from the corners of the eyes, on the edges of the bones of the eye sockets on the side of the head)

tf tiny **f**inger (beside the nail on the side toward the thumb)

un under **n**ose (below the nose on the upper lip)

ch chin (in the cleft between the chin and lower lip)

g gamut spot (on the back of the hand in the indentation between the bones of the tiny finger and the ring finger about ½ inch back onto the hand—use [2 OR 3] fingers to tap)

9g 9 Gamut Sequence—Tap the gamut spot continuously while doing the following:

1. Close the eyes
2. Open the eyes

3. Move the eyes down and to one side
4. Move the eyes down and to other side
5. Roll the eyes in a circle in one direction
6. Roll the eyes in a circle in the opposite direction
7. Hum a tune (about five notes) out loud with mouth closed
8. Count aloud from one to five
9. Hum a tune again aloud, with mouth closed

er floor-to-ceiling **eye r**oll (while tapping the gamut spot, hold head level. Move eyes. Look down to the floor, and slowly, to a count of 10, slowly roll your eyes vertically up to the ceiling).

If Individual Energy Toxins Interfere with an Algorithm Treatment

The following suggestions are provided as a means to attempt to deal with treatments that don't work, often due to Individual Energy Toxins (IETs), which keep the algorithm from being effective. Use these only when you are comfortable to continue.

What To Do If A Treatment Doesn't Work

TFT algorithms have a remarkably high success rate; however, there will be people who will not be able to get the desired result at the algorithm level. If you have been through the steps of an algorithm and the SUD remains unchanged, first consult this book to ensure that you actually did each step correctly.

Ask yourself:

- Did I do the correct sequence for the appropriate algorithm?
- Did I remember to do the PR reversal correction and then repeat the treatment?
- Have I tried using any alternative algorithms listed in the book for the problem being addressed?
- Have I tried doing the collarbone breathing treatment?

Important:

One common error that people make is to repeat an algorithm that didn't work. If it didn't work on the first try after going through all the steps in their proper sequence (including PR correction and CB2), it will not help to repeat the treatment. This will only result in frustration.

At this point, you should do a further assessment in order to determine if there are other associated aspects of the problem that need to be addressed with other algorithms. If so, do them using the same steps as outlined in the TFT protocol.

You can also ask yourself if you are still thinking about the problem in the same way as you were when you started the treatment. It is possible that the original thought field has been eliminated, and that you are in a new thought field.

If you suspect that you have been exposed to a toxin, try the following:

- Tap the index finger about 15 times, and then tap the PR spot (side of hand) 15 times. Now, immediately repeat the Algorithm which did not seem to help and see if the same treatment will work now.

Other things to do:

- Open a window or door to freshen the air.
- Change location—try out of doors (fresh air vs. air conditioning).
- Change into clothing that has been cleaned in a different manner.
- Wrap a clean towel or surgical (paper) gown over offending clothing.
- Wash off any scented cosmetics, perfume, or after shave lotion.
- Wear a medical mask.

- Attempt to dilute the toxin. Have the client drink a large glass of filtered water and wait a few minutes.
- Wait for a few minutes. This is not such a quick fix; however, it can sometimes make a difference.
- Return at another time wearing no cosmetics, no perfume, having not smoked, etc.

If you have followed the procedures for all aspects of the problem and still have no change, the next step is to call an algorithm instructor or other practitioner who is trained at TFT Diagnostic level or higher. Details can be obtained from the web sites, **www. tftrx.com** and **www.atft.org,** or by speaking to a customer service representative in the Callahan Techniques, Ltd. office.

Contact details are given at the back of this book.

You can also obtain the Toxin Kit from Callahan Techniques, Ltd. This contains audiotapes and videotapes to assist you in diagnosing and treating toxins.

The exception to this is the addiction algorithm, which commonly needs to be repeated every time the client gets the urge for what he/she is addicted to.

Identifying Individual Energy Toxins

Method 1—Find patterns linked to exposure.

When a TFT cure has been undone and your level of distress goes back up while you are in the ***original*** Thought Field, you have probably been exposed to an IET. Please note that thought fields may change.

- Ask yourself what you have eaten or inhaled prior to the return of the problem.
- Look for the patterns in your psychological and physical responses to exposures.

- On bad days or moments, track what you have eaten or inhaled.
- Keep a journal to record daily exposures and a food diary that includes symptoms.

Method 2—Use Coca's Pulse Test.

Dr. Coca's book, *The Pulse Test*, provides extensive background information and instruction for using this method.

- Find a baseline pulse, and compare this with the pulse immediately after exposure to a potential toxin and up to an hour later.
- A resting heart rate of more than 84 beats per minute usually indicates that the person has been exposed to an IET.
- An increase in pulse rate of more than a few beats per minute after exposure to a toxin will also indicate sensitivity.
- A difference of over 10 beats per minute between sitting and standing will indicate the presence of a toxin.

Addictive Urges and the Anxiety / Addiction Connection

In my book, *The Anxiety Addiction Connection: Eliminate your Addictive Urges with TFT* (1995), I explain that the growing problem of addiction is due to the prevalence of the problem of anxiety. I propose that all addictions are attempts to reduce anxiety, although the addictive substances and behaviours actually only serve to **mask** the anxiety and **do nothing** to eliminate it.

Therefore, addiction is tied to anxiety as an associated response. In fact, it is often the only conscious response. The anxiety itself is apparently out of the addict's awareness until the craving returns. Rather than consciously feeling the anxiety, the person becomes aware of a craving for the addictive substance (or behaviour). Anytime you feel anxious about anything, treat it, and notice how much more smoothly your life goes. You may notice health benefits and an improved quality of life, as well.

That is, any time you feel any of the areas we have described above as a reason to eat when you are **not** hungry, treat yourself with the anxiety or cravings algorithm and notice just how much better you feel about yourself.

A practical example of the Anxiety Algorithm

Using the treatment points on the chart seen earlier we are now going to practice the algorithm for anxiety.

1. Tune into the feeling of anxiety and
2. Identify the level of anxiety (SUD) on a scale of 1 to 10
3. Tap 5 times under the eye
4. Tap 5 times under the arm
5. Tap 5 times on the collarbone
6. Identify the current SUD
7. If the SUD is 5 or less go to number 9
8. If the SUD is above 5 repeat 3 – 5 until it is 5 or less.
9. Carry out the 9g process
10. If SUD is 2 or less carry out the Eye Roll
11. If SUD is greater than 2 treat for PR and repeat the majors and 9G treatment until SUD is 2 or less.

Using the treatment points on the chart seen earlier we are now going to practice the algorithm for addictive urges and cravings.

1. Tune into the feeling of addictive urge or craving and
2. Identify the level of addictive urge or craving (SUD) on a scale of 1 to 10
3. Tap 5 times on the collarbone
4. Tap 5 times under the eye
5. Tap 5 times on the collarbone
6. Identify the current SUD
7. If the SUD is 5 or less go to number
8. If the SUD is above 5 repeat 3 – 5 until it is 5 or less.

9   Carry out the 9g process

10   If SUD is 2 or less carry out the Eye Roll

11   If SUD is greater than 2 treat for PR and repeat the majors and 9G treatment until SUD is 2 or less.

The algorithm for addictive urge and craving is not a one-off cure. You will need to repeat it for every urge or craving as they occur until you lose the craving.

You now have all you need to understand TFT in principle and to be able to treat yourself and your loved ones for basic anxiety and cravings.

I wish you every success in the future

Dr Roger Callahan
Creator of Thought Field Therapy®

For more information on how to obtain further help or instruction please visit www.tftrx.com and www.oh-crikey,.com

Appendix 2
Maximum Heart Rate measurement

Firstly, make sure you warm up properly before doing any exercise.

Find a step of about 8 inches in height. Begin a four count and on 1 step up with your right leg on 2 bring your left leg up on 3 your right leg down and on 4 your left leg down. Do this roughly every 2 seconds for 3 minutes. That is 90 times. Measure your heart rate at the end of the 3 minutes.

Now assess your fitness factor. Are you really fit (65 points) or in excellent condition (55 points) or average (45 points) or poor (35 points). Be honest and then add these points to your hear rate. That is your step factor.

Now when you are back at rest, sit on a chair. Stand up and sit down every two seconds for 3 minutes. Ninety times and then measure your heart rate. Add your fitness factor points to your heart rate like this. Fit add 80, excellent add 70, average add 60 and poor add 50.

Add your two factors together and divide by two to get your suggested maximum heart rate. For example:

Step final heart rate = 120   Fitness level = average = 45
Total = 165   Chair final heart rate = 115
Fitness level = average = 60   Total = 175

Suggested Maximum Heart Rate = 165 + 175 = 240 / 2 = **170 beats per minute**

Appendix 3
Standard Algorithms for use with Weight Management

This section provide you with the standard algorithms for common issues and then adds some variations for you to use in the standard algorithm does not produce the desired effect. Standard algorithms are effective normally for 80% of people. If you have continuing issues with lowering your SUD, it may be advantageous to visit a TFT practitioner near you for diagnosis. You may find a suitable practitioner (they will have trained to Diagnosis levels I & II) on the ATFT website at www.atft.org and look under Membership Directory.

Algorithms

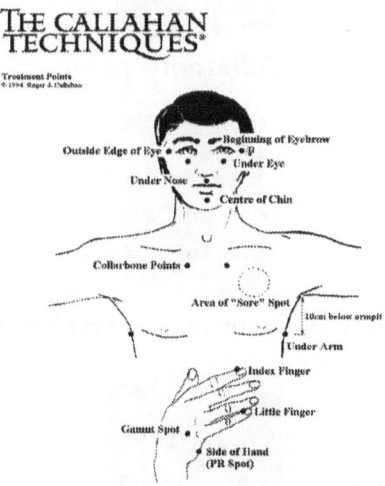

THE CALLAHAN TECHNIQUES®

Treatment Points
© 1994 Roger J. Callahan

Beginning of Eyebrow
Outside Edge of Eye
Under Eye
Under Nose
Centre of Chin
Collarbone Points
Area of "Sore" Spot
10cm below armpit
Under Arm
Index Finger
Little Finger
Gamut Spot
Side of Hand
(PR Spot)

Key to letters

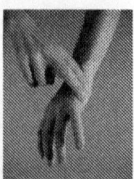

soh (PR spot) - Side of hand

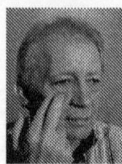

e - Under the eye

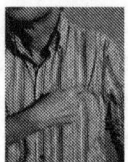

a - Under the arm

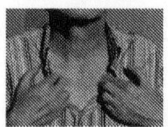

c - Collarbone point

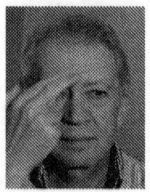

eb - Beginning of Eyebrow (nearest bridge of nose)

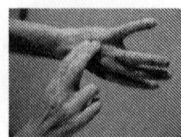

9g - 9 Gamut sequence

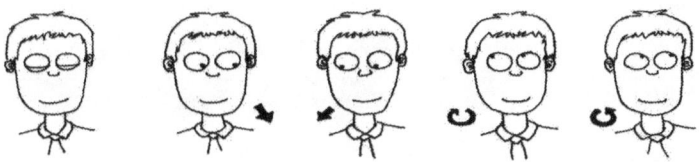

sq - Repeat the sequence of Majors

er - Floor to ceiling eye roll.

Algorithm sequences

Anxiety   e, a, c, 9g, sq, er

Addiction/Craving   e, c, a, c, 9g, sq, er
             Or   c, a, c, 9g, sq, er
             Or   a, e, c, 9g, sq, er

Panic/Anxiety   eb, e, a, c, 9g, sq, er
                        c, a, eb, c, 9g, sq, er
                        a, e, eb, c, 9g, sq, er

Inability to visualise a, c, 9g, sq, er

Self sabotage   Correct for PR. Side of Hand 15 times

I have included the ER (Eye Roll in the above algorithms but this should only be used once your SUD has reached 2 or less).

There are many more standard algorithms for a wide variety of issues. These can be learned by attending a formal TFT training course and learning how to apply the therapy accurately in all situations. Courses can found by emailing info@oh-crikey.com and there are lists of courses on www.atft.org and www.tftrx.com

www.ingramcontent.com/pod-product-compliance
Lightning Source LLC
Chambersburg PA
CBHW061254280526
45784CB00002B/763